Professional Issues and Ethics in Physical Therapy

T0266288

Professional Issues and Ethics in Physical Therapy

A Case-Based Approach

Second Edition

NANCY R. KIRSCH, PT, DPT, PhD, FAPTA

Vice Chair Rehabilitation and Movement Sciences
Professor, Doctor of Physical Therapy Program
School of Health Professions
Rutgers, The State University of New Jersey
New Brunswick, New Jersey

New York   Chicago   San Francisco   London   Madrid   Mexico City
Milan   New Delhi   Singapore   Sydney   Toronto

Professional Issues and Ethics in Physical Therapy: A Case-Based Approach, Second Edition

1 2 3 4 5 6 7 8 9 LCR 28 27 26 25 24 23

ISBN: 978-1-264-28542-6
MHID: 1-264-28542-6

This book was set in Minion Pro by MPS Limited.
The editors were Sydney Keen Vitale and Christina M. Thomas.
The production supervisor was Richard Ruzycka.
Project management was provided by Himanshu Abrol, MPS Limited.
The cover designer was W2 Design.

Library of Congress Control Number: 2023940742

Dedication

To my husband Shel and my loving immediate and extended family,
who give me space to continue to learn, evolve, and develop
but are always there to support me, encourage me, and
"welcome me home."

My students of over 30 years who give me hope for
our future as a profession.

My colleagues at Rutgers University
who embody professionalism and ethical wisdom.

Eric Ries, associate editor of APTA's PT in Motion,
for his constant wisdom and guidance.

Most importantly, to my patients,
who for the past half century have given meaning to my life
as they have invited me to be part of theirs.

Contents

Foreword

Thousands of physical therapists, physical therapist assistants, and students have benefited from the "ethical lens" provided by the ethics column written by Nancy Kirsch, PT, DPT, PhD, FAPTA, and published in PT in Motion. This series of ethics articles was a constant reminder to the physical therapy community about the ethical dimension of physical therapy practice in every setting. Ethical issues in physical therapy range from relatively simple challenges of courteous professional behavior and communication to vexing dilemmas between competing ethical obligations and confusing situations of moral ambiguity.

Dr. Kirsch's ongoing work through publication and professional presentations has elevated our profession's understanding of ethical issues in physical therapy. This new book continues this "moral dialogue" with the physical therapy community. The case studies draw on Dr. Kirsch's wealth of professional experience and wisdom gained as a practitioner, educator, and leader in physical therapy. The importance of case deliberation in the development of moral reasoning skills has been well established; and this book can be an important tool for students and practitioners in honing ethical reasoning skills. Dr. Kirsch's ability to create real-life, practical, and engaging cases will be appreciated by students, educators, and clinicians frustrated by hypothetical cases that may miss the mark. I have no doubt that this book will become a trusted professional resource for students, educators, and practitioners confronting ethical issues in daily practice.

Laura Lee (Dolly) Swisher, PT, PhD, FNAP, FAPTA

Preface

Over the past century in the United States, physical therapy evolved from a technical field to a doctoring profession. This evolution reflects significant growth in the body of knowledge that a clinician must acquire and apply. What is even more significant than the growth in technical skills is the demands of professional behavior that the practice of physical therapy now requires. When physical therapists worked under the direction of another health care provider, the ethical decisions they were faced with making were often seemingly out of their control. Decisions about patient care and access to care were not only influenced by others but controlled by other than the treating physical therapist. The changes in the profession are reflected in the changes in the Code of Ethics that provides guidance to practicing PT's. The very first Code of Ethics introduced early in the development of the profession addressed primarily the individual realm, our relationship with our patients and the relationship with our colleagues. The revisions of the Code that occurred during the next several decades did not change this frame of reference very much. As a nascent profession PT was very inwardly focused and the patient–therapist relationship was of course the center of that focus. Subsequent revisions of the Code and Standards mirrored the change in the profession as direct access became accepted across the jurisdictions, and PTs were educated in all CAPTE accredited programs at the Doctoral level. Ethical dialogue among colleagues resulting in identification of professional challenges and discussion of action plans is critically important to moving our profession forward and to empowering every PT and PTA to "own their own practice."

The very nature of physical therapy, the close physical and personal connection between PTs and their patients makes the discipline one that is often perched precariously on the slippery slope of boundary violations, dual relationships, institutional and supervisory power gradient challenges and a host of other potential difficult situations. For over fifteen years the professional association dedicated space monthly for the discussion of ethical issues that apply to all clinicians regardless of setting or field of practice. This text was designed to give practical ethics a home, to provide tools that both students and clinicians could easily use to become facile in managing ethical challenges in practice. The cases are set up to encourage discussion. The text provides a framework to answer the "should" questions. What should I do? How should I act? The format provides the opportunity to move beyond the individual realm, when appropriate, resolving issues within an institutional or societal perspective.

This text is divided into two separate and discreet sections. They are designed to integrate with one another, but each section can also be used separately. Physical therapy ethics is a dynamic and evolving field of study and a constantly changing part of clinical practice. Practical guidance is often best incorporated into practice through activities that involve dialogue between clinicians and though this book is focused on physical therapy cases they are real world situations that are appropriate for a multidisciplinary discussion.

The purpose of this text is to give students and clinicians a lens through which to analyze contemporary ethical challenges. Philosophical theory within the text is limited to that which can be applied practically in the clinical setting. A suggested model for ethical decision-making is introduced and applied but it is not the only way in which to approach and resolve ethical situations. Ethical decision making is a component of clinical decision-making and they share to an extent reasonable ambiguity. The challenge for all of us to become comfortable and confident in working with an amount of uncertainty. The question always arises "can we teach somebody to be ethical." This text is not a primer on ethical behavior. It is designed to provide students and clinicians with a framework in which to approach the uncertainty of ethical decision making with tools to aid their inherent good judgment. Discussions of professional issues, the "What should I do?" questions are stimulating and force us to reach into the depths of our reasoning acumen. It is hoped that whether you use this text as a future physical therapist, a clinician, or an educator, you will appreciate the privilege we have as healthcare providers to engage in these professional discussions that improve the lives of our patients and encourage us to continue to do what is right, what is responsible, and what leads to consistent safe and effective clinical practice.

How to Use This Book

There are two parts to this book. Part One provides more didactic, foundational material while Part Two strives to apply ethical decision making tools to relevant cases in physical therapy practice. The two parts are meant to be used together but they also can stand alone providing basic conceptual material about ethics, and ethical decision-making in physical therapy practice, with the second section focusing on case analysis.

This text begins with foundational material that serves as a good introduction for students and a light review for practicing clinicians. Each chapter in the first section of the text concludes with *Ideas to Consider.* **Chapter One** introduces the reader to healthcare ethics with a brief overview of how ethical decision making has evolved. It is not the intention of the book to make the reader a bioethicist. Rather the chapter introduces the terms utilized in the field of Bioethics with the clinical relevance highlighted with references to the Code of Ethics to provide a practical application of the term. The chapter also gives us insight into the responsibility we have to take action, exercise moral potency, not to be passive in the relationship that benefits those who have entrusted their care to us. The chapter concludes with a brief discussion of the relationship between ethics and law. **Chapter Two** explores the evolution of the Code of Ethics for the Physical Therapists and the Standards of Ethical Conduct for the Physical Therapist Assistant. It focuses on how these core documents and our core values have evolved as the profession of physical therapy has evolved. It is meant to provide a strong framework for clinicians to rely on to empower them to work collaboratively but to accept the challenge and the imperative to take personal responsibility for sound professional judgments. **Chapter Three** establishes the framework of professionalism and sets the foundation for ethical decision making firmly on the patient/therapist relationship, the importance of trust and the dynamic involved in that trust are developed in this chapter. **Chapter Four,** ethical guidance can stand alone, independent of any other aspect of the text but it is also a foundation to understanding how we as physical therapists and physical therapist assistants are expected to behave. It delves into each of the principles and standards of the Code of Ethics for the physical therapist and the Standards of Ethical Conduct of the physical therapist assistant. Regardless of role, to work together effectively, the PT and the PTA must understand their ethical obligations as well as the ethical obligations of their colleagues. **Chapter Five,** ethical risk factors, addresses the "unthinkable" the fact that any one of us can easily engage in an ethical breach, because just like our patients we are human and not infallible. This chapter lends itself to an opportunity for introspection, how many of the risk factors identified have I had in the past, or currently have or may have in the future, suggestions are offered for how to recognize potential risks, and how to mitigate those risks if possible. A new section has been added to this chapter addressing the concept of moral injury, and how a clinician suffering from moral injury is more likely to have a negative impact on a patient.

Chapter Six is the heart of the ethical decision-making portion of the text and if you are planning to use just the cases, you would benefit from first reviewing Chapter Six to provide the context for efficient ways in which to utilize the suggested decision-making model. Two cases are presented and developed fully to model an extensive ethical decision-making framework. When using the cases in Part Two it is often helpful to return to this chapter to review application of the decision-making frameworks. Ethical decision-making is what is expected of professionals by the public we are privileged to work with. The complications in ethical decision-making arise not just from the individual relationships we have with patients but on the confounding factors that develop because of the influences of the institutions and organizations and the societal pressures that impact our practice. With each passing day, and each technological advance, the questions become more complex impacted by resource allocation, access to PT services, and technological advances. This chapter poses the question that we are consistently faced with ... "just because we can, doesn't mean we should." **Chapter Seven** is new to the second edition, reflecting dramatic practice changes that evolved over the past few years in telehealth and digital physical therapy practice. The first edition addresses telehealth in the ethical challenges of the future chapter but the future is now, and telehealth and digital health both have notable advantages for patient care but at the same time raise interesting ethical questions. **Chapter Eight** is also new to the second edition and is a result of that all-important clinical dialogue. Clinicians began to notice a significant uptick in questions from patients and clinicians and students about verbal, nonverbal, and even physical behaviors that appeared to cross the line between appropriate and less than appropriate behavior. What does the PT clinician, educator, researcher, administrator need to be aware of when practicing a hands-on profession in a hands-off world? The final chapter in Part One, **Chapter Nine** looks to the future, that which challenges us today will always be just a part of what will challenge us tomorrow and as professionals we have an obligation not just to keep up with new advances clinically but also with the new ethical challenges that arise from the technological changes.

Part Two of the text is designed to be integrated with Part One or it can stand alone for clinical or class discussions. The cases are divided into the major areas in which ethical decisions fall in clinical practice. Each section now has four cases with a new case added for each section related to updated material presented in section one on this second edition. When used in a clinical setting, cases can be used independently to encourage discussion or to stimulate thought as background for a clinically relevant case in the setting in which you are practicing. In the classroom setting the four cases per section allow you many options about how to use the cases either in a dedicated ethics or professional issues class or to integrate the cases into clinical courses as they may be applicable to that course content. You can use one case to introduce the process in the classroom and then use subsequent cases for either individual work to be discussed in class or group work.

Chapter Ten provides an introduction to case analysis guiding the reader through a case with suggestions on how the case analysis process could be applied. **Chapter Eleven** deals with cases having to do with professional accountability, particularly when the PT is navigating the many entities to whom they are accountable to. **Chapter Twelve** navigates the always tricky area of boundary issues. In a profession that gets so close to their patients physically and emotionally boundary awareness is critical and boundary breeches always a concern. **Chapter Thirteen** covers the broad spectrum of practice issues. PT's treat across the lifespan, in a myriad of practice settings and each situation is unique but the basic responsibilities of the physical therapist remain constant regardless of setting or patient presentation. This chapter is focused on helping the PT drill down to the core parameters of ethical practice. **Chapter Fourteen** traverses the complex but critical area of professional relationships both intra professional and inter professional both critical to maintaining a productive working environment. The cases speak to the carefully traversed path between the necessity to be autonomous in our decision-making but at the same time be collaborative and not isolated in our practice. **Chapter Fifteen** addresses professional responsibility. This complex relationship that we have with all the institutions that impact our practice is most important to understand in the context of our responsibility to our colleagues, profession, and most important our patients. The cases in this chapter explore professional responsibility from various perspectives. **Chapter Sixteen** addresses self-regulation, every professional has the responsibility to regulate themselves as well as the responsibility to be accountable for the regulation of physical therapy practice. The public grants professionals the right to regulate their own practice and with that comes the responsibility of professionals to be deliberate and thoughtful about what that privilege/responsibility requires. **Chapter Seventeen** traverses the complex world of supervision and being supervised. It is built on the premise that *delegation does not mean abdication*. These cases look at the responsibility of the supervisor as well as the responsibility of the person being supervised. The ultimate responsibility whether supervisor or supervisee lies with the individual licensee, often leading to some very complicated ethical situations. **Chapter Eighteen,** the final chapter in the book navigates the very special relationship between the novice, the student physical therapist, and their future profession. There is a uniqueness to healthcare education that requires a considerable amount of on-the-job training as part of the formal education. This training, while highly beneficial, places unique and complex responsibilities on both the student and the licensed clinician. Many of the issues discussed in previous chapters impact the student, clinical instructor relationship but there are some situations that are unique to this very special student, teacher, mentor, future colleague relationship.

The challenge of this text is to constantly keep it relevant and current providing new cases via on line resources that reflect new professional challenges, but the text itself with its foundation in principle and application should endure and provide continued meaning and relevance to inform clinical practice and encourage practitioners to consistently to strive to do what is right recognizing that there is never a "right way" to do the "wrong thing."

Professional Issues and Ethics in Physical Therapy

PART ONE

Ethics for the Physical Therapist

CHAPTER 1

Healthcare Ethics

Reports of ethics violations in government, industry, and the financial world have captured the attention of the public in recent times. The omnipresent nature of today's news media contributes to the revelation of misdoings in a way never seen before. In every sector of the economy, ethical violations make news. In medicine, the topic of ethics evolved slowly from the 2500-year-old Oath of Hippocrates over many centuries to the biomedical ethics of today (Edelstein, 1967; Sugarman, 2000). The body of knowledge around ethical theory is evolving rapidly now, fed by challenges that the healthcare delivery system places on practitioners as well as significant changes in healthcare that present new challenges for providers such as the use of digital healthcare data (Aicardi et al., 2016; Kirsch, 2017; Means et al., 2015; Pasztor, 2015; Wells et al., 2015).

Society demands exceptional behavior from its healthcare practitioners, and currently, there is increased awareness when ethical breaches occur as well as renewed expectation of a high level of ethical behavior (Tenery, 2016). Physical therapists (PTs) often find themselves at the forefront of ethical decision-making. Because it is not possible to behave ethically without a thorough understanding of the standards of practice for one's own healthcare field, this book is designed to help clinicians to utilize guidelines for making good ethical decisions in physical therapy practice (Dubois, 2018, Marques, 2012; Quigley, 2015).

Healthcare providers recognize they are entrusted with a special relationship with their patients, one based on trust. This is one of the pillars of professionalism, which is the foundation of the societal contract (Cruess, 2006). Healthcare providers have a special fiduciary responsibility to patients who generally have an injury or disability providing special challenges because of their increased vulnerability within the general population. Yet, even though PTs understand the need to make ethics-based clinical decisions, their ethical decision-making skills may be under-developed (Hudon et al., 2015; Naamanka et al., 2020; Strum, 2023). All physical therapy providers are faced with the challenges of a swiftly changing medical environment that includes redefining of roles, advances in education, and increases in the scope and nature of practice, all factors that challenge professional behaviors and require the education and training to manage the ethical decision-making that is always integral to clinical decision-making (Brody and Doukas, 2014; Miles and Prasad, 2016; Murrell, 2014).

PTs are generally independent professionals delivering services directly to patients. In addition, the entry-level education of PTs in the United States is the clinical doctorate. As of 2017 all CAPTE-accredited schools require that the Doctor of Physical Therapy be the entry-level degree (CAPTE, 2016). This raises public expectations of the level of practice of a PT. The public's demand for transparency and the growing visibility of other healthcare providers have increased the pressure on all health providers and other non-physicians to be more accountable for their actions. Pellegrino (1999) refers to physical therapy as a "relatively new" profession, one in which "ethical maturity has not yet completely evolved." That statement, over 20 years ago in some respects, is still true as PTs struggle with ethical decision-making in many clinical situations (Hightower and Klinker, 2012; Hudon et al., 2015).

Dove (1995) speaks of the loss of trust the public has in professionals in the helping fields and how the loss of trust can be prevented with appropriate education in professional ethics (Sokol, 2015; Strum, 2023; Sutherland-Smith and Saltmarsh, 2011). This requires that knowledge of ethical behavior by clinicians be disseminated to the public to help maintain and, if necessary, restore trust. It is critical that this begins in the entry-level education program where breaches of ethical behavior are not tolerated (Dar and Kahn, 2021; deOliveira et al., 2015; Nijhof et al., 2012; Pantic and Wubbels, 2012; Rawson et al., 2013).

Scott (1998) reasoned that loyalty to the patient can be very difficult to reconcile with the organizational priorities and financial pressures associated with care today. PTs have a fiduciary (financial) obligation toward their patients. PTs and physical therapist assistants (PTAs) are today confronted with ethical situations in which it has become increasingly difficult to deliver care effectively (Balak et al., 2020). For example, in a 2003 study of more than 450 practicing PTs, 64% of the respondents felt that the number of ethical issues confronting PTs in the past 10 years had increased, and 97% felt they either stayed the same or increased. Fewer than 2% of the respondents felt the number of issues decreased (Kirsch, 2003). These findings are consistent with those in other health fields (Balak et al., 2020; Hightower and Klinker, 2012; Kaldjian et al., 2013).

The responsibility of a profession to manage its own ethical "house" was identified over 40 years ago. Andrew Guccione (1980) stated: "The need to identify and clarify ethical issues within physical therapy increases as the profession assumes responsibility for those areas of direct care in its domain." Susan Sisola further identified the responsibility of practitioners, stating: "The privilege and influence that accompany professional practice obligate healthcare providers to look beyond literal or superficial interpretations of their ethical code, and to consider the complexities of the ethical issues evident in the current practice environment" (Avey et al., 2009; Avolio et al., 2009; Balak et al., 2020; Hannah et al., 2008; Knapp et al., 2013a, 2013b; Sisola, 2003)

Healthcare ethics are unique. The expectations are higher for healthcare providers because patients often cannot choose who they want as a healthcare provider. They are vulnerable to variations in care and to potential exploitation, and the result of poor behavior on the part of the practitioner can have dire consequences not just for the patient but for the reputation of the profession (Barnett et al., 2005; Caldicott and D'Oronzio, 2014; Hren et al., 2011; Mansbach et al., 2012).

THE LANGUAGE OF BIOETHICS

Like any other body of knowledge, it is important to correctly use the terminology specific to the area of study so that there is little question on what the intent is. A common error in discussing ethical issues is to call them all a dilemma, but as we will discuss in Chapter 6, the Chapter about ethical decision making, a dilemma refers only to a specific type of ethical situation in which the potential courses of action could all be correct. The language of biomedical ethics is applied across all practice settings, and four basic principles are commonly accepted by bioethicists. These principles include (1) autonomy, (2) beneficence, (3) nonmaleficence, and (4) justice. In physical therapy, and other health fields, veracity and fidelity are also spoken of as ethical principles, but they are not part of the foundational ethical principles identified by bioethicists.

One of the most confusing aspects of navigating through ethical conversations is clearly expressing what we are talking about and what we are basing our ethical decision-making upon:

Ethical Principles: The four basic principles that ethical decision-making uses as a foundation are autonomy, beneficence, nonmaleficence, and justice. For our purposes we will also include veracity and fidelity.

Code of Ethics Principles: The APTA Code of Ethics contains eight principles, and within those eight there are another 38 principles that provide the practicing PT with clear guidance in managing ethical issues (APTA, 2017a).

Standards of Ethical Conduct: The APTA Standards of Ethical Conduct mirror in many ways the topic areas addressed in the Code of Ethics but are specifically intended to guide the work that the PTA does (APTA, 2017b).

Core Values: The core values are linked to the Code of Ethics and the Standards of Ethical Conduct; they also provide guidance to the clinician on how to manage an ethical issue. We will explore the application of these different tools in Chapter 5 when we look at various ethical decision-making processes. The American Physical Therapy Association identifies the following as core values for the profession: accountability, altruism, collaboration, compassion/caring, excellence, integrity, professional duty, social responsibility.

The Principle of Autonomy

Autonomy is an American value. We espouse great respect for individual rights and equate freedom with autonomy. Our system of law supports autonomy and, as a corollary, upholds the right of individuals to make decisions about their own healthcare.

Respect for autonomy requires that patients be told the truth about their condition and informed about the risk and benefits of treatment. Under the law, they are permitted to refuse treatment even if the best and most reliable information indicates that treatment would be beneficial, unless their action may have a negative impact on the well-being of another individual. These conflicts set the stage for ethical dilemmas, where two courses of action may be correct.

The concept of autonomy has evolved from paternalistic physicians who held ethical decision-making authority, to patients empowered to participate in making decisions about their own care, to patients heavily armed with Internet resources who seek to prevail in any decision making. This transition of authority has been slower to evolve in the geriatric population, but as the baby boomers age, they will assert this evolving standard of independence. Autonomy, however, does not negate responsibility. Healthcare is at its foundation a partnership between the provider and the recipient of care. Each owes the other responsibility and respect (Kilic et al., 2021; Veatch, 2016).

CLINICAL RELEVANCE

Physical therapists have as one of their five roles the obligation to teach. This is particularly relevant to the concept of autonomy as educating a patient provides them with the tools to make an informed decision regarding their care. This is consistent with Principles 2C and 2D of the Code of Ethics: **2C:** Physical therapists shall provide the information necessary to allow patients or their surrogates to make informed decisions about physical therapy care or participation in clinical research. **2D:** Physical therapists shall collaborate with patients/clients to empower them in decisions about their healthcare.

The Principle of Beneficence

The beneficent practitioner provides care that is in the best interest of the patient. **Beneficence** is the act of being kind. The actions of the healthcare provider are designed to bring about a positive good. Beneficence always raises the question of subjective and objective determinations of benefit versus harm. A beneficent decision can only be objective if the same decision was made regardless of who was making it. The idea of beneficence is steeped in the concept of care and concern, and it is one of the foundational pillars of the patient/therapist relationship. Inherent in the role of a healthcare provider is the desire to be beneficent, yet how the provider sees their actions and how the patient interprets the actions can be significantly different. It is not uncommon for an act of beneficence thought to be in the best interest of the individual to come into conflict with the patient's desire for a different action that they express through their autonomy.

Traditionally, the ethical decision-making process and the ultimate decision were the purview of the physician. This is no longer the case; the patient and other health-care providers, according to their specific expertise, are central to the decision-making process (Valente and Saunders, 2000). For example, physical and occupational therapists have expertise in quality-of-life issues, and in this capacity can offer much to the discussions of lifestyle and life-challenging choices, particularly when dealing with terminal diseases and end-of-life situations (Leeuwenburgh-Pronk et al., 2015). PTs as movement specialists have a unique perspective on the interaction of all the systems in the body to elicit movement. The PTs have the responsibility to always place the patient at the center of the decision-making process, cognizant of the confounding institutional and societal factors that may influence the decisions they make.

CLINICAL RELEVANCE

Physical therapists have as one of their five roles patient/client management. This is particularly relevant to the concept of beneficence as the patient remains central to the idea of caring. This is consistent with many principles, which we will explore later in case studies, but the overarching theme is Principles 1A, 2A, and 2B of the Code of Ethics: **1A:** Physical therapists shall act in a respectful manner toward each person regardless of age, gender, race, nationality, religion, ethnicity, social or economic status, sexual orientation, health condition, or disability. **2A:** Physical therapists shall adhere to the core values of the profession and shall act in the best interests of patients/clients over the interests of the physical therapists. **2B:** Physical therapists shall provide physical therapy services with compassionate and caring behaviors that incorporate the individual and cultural differences of patients/clients.

The Principle of Nonmaleficence

Nonmaleficence means doing no harm. Providers must ask themselves whether their actions may harm the patient either by omission or commission. The guiding principle of *primum non nocere*, "first of all, do no harm," is based in the Hippocratic Oath. Actions or practices of a healthcare provider are "right" as long as they are in the interest of the patient and avoid negative consequences. There is often confusion between the two principles of beneficence and nonmaleficence. If a practitioner is beneficent then they could not possibly cause harm, yet they can. The two principles are distinct and require the practitioner to consider both.

The question is always appropriate to ask, "In my desire to be beneficent could I potentially either knowingly or unwittingly be harming the patient?" Another question that we must always ask ourselves is "Just because we can ... should we?" This query often arises when dealing with end-of-life issues. We have, with the help of medical technology, the ability to prolong life ... which is in juxtaposition to the ability to allow death to occur. Both have elements of overt action and deliberate inaction.

Patients with terminal illnesses are often concerned that technology will maintain their life beyond their wishes; thus, healthcare providers are challenged to improve care during this end stage of life. Patients may even choose to hasten death if options are available (Phipps et al., 2003). The right of the individual to choose to "die with dignity" is the ultimate manifestation of autonomy, but it is difficult for healthcare providers to accept death when there may still be viable options. Here we see the principle of nonmaleficence conflicting with the principle of autonomy as the desire of healthcare providers to be beneficent or, at the least, cause no harm may conflict with the choice of the patient. The active choice to hasten death versus the seemingly passive choice of allowing death to occur requires that we provide patients with all the information necessary to make an informed choice about courses of action available to them.

A complicating factor in end-of-life decisions is the patients' concern that, even if they make their wishes clear (e.g., through an advance directive), their family members or surrogates will not be able to carry out their desires and permit death to occur (Phipps et al., 2003). Treating against the wishes of the patient can potentially result in mental anguish and subsequent harm for all parties involved.

CLINICAL RELEVANCE

This principle, which is similar to the principle of beneficence, is consistent with the patient/client management role. The patient remains central to the idea of caring and not causing harm. With the patient as the central focus, Principles 3A, 3B, and 3C of the Code of Ethics should be considered: **3A:** Physical therapists shall demonstrate independent and objective professional judgment in the patient's/client's best interest in all practice settings. **3B:** Physical therapists shall demonstrate professional judgment informed by professional standards, evidence (including current literature and established best practice), practitioner experience, and patient/client values. **3C:** Physical therapists shall make judgments within their scope of practice and level of expertise and shall communicate with, collaborate with, or refer to peers or other healthcare professionals when necessary.

The Principle of Justice

Justice speaks to equity and fairness in treatment. Hippocrates related ethical principles to the individual relationship between the physician and the patient. Ethical theory today must extend beyond individuals to the institutional and societal realms (Gabard and Martin, 2003).

Justice may be seen as having two types: distributive and comparative. **Distributive justice** addresses the degree to which healthcare services are distributed equitably throughout society. Within the logic of distributive justice, we should treat similar cases similarly, but how can we determine if cases are indeed similar?

Looking at the principles of justice as they relate to the delivery of care, it is apparent that they do conflict in many circumstances; for example, a real-life system that attempts to provide an equal share to each person is distributing resources that are not without limit. When good patient care demands more than the system has allocated, there may be a need for adjustments within the marketplace. The concept of justice which often demands that we allocate resources is often a source of conflicting choices for practitioners.

Comparative justice determines how healthcare is delivered at the individual level. It looks at disparate treatment of patients on the basis of age, disability, gender, race, ethnicity, and religion. Of particular interest currently are the disparities that occur because of age. In 1975, Singer related bias as a result of age to gender and race discrimination and referred to the practice as **ageism** (Gabard and Martin, 2003). In a society where equal access to healthcare does not exist, there is a continuing concern about the distribution of resources, particularly as the population ages and the demand for services increases. What will the burdens on the system cause? How do we manage to allocate resources that are not without limit, including human capital, time, and money?

The first wave of baby boomers is receiving Medicare, and the health spending projections for the next decade are significant (Keehan et al., 2008). Thorpe and Howard (2006) found that there has been an increase in medication use of 11.5% in the past decade just for the medical management of metabolic syndrome, an age-associated complex of diseases. McWilliams and colleagues (2007) found that Medicare beneficiaries who were previously uninsured, and who enrolled in Medicare at age 65, may have greater morbidity, requiring more intensive and costlier care, than they would have had had they been previously insured. The cost to the system of low levels of care is extensive. As the number of Americans who had very poor insurance or were uninsured will ultimately come into the Medicare program with potentially greater morbidity, the demands of justice in the healthcare system will continue to increase. Approximately 15% of the U.S. population is enrolled in the Medicare program. Enrollment is expected to rise to 79 million by 2030 (Kaiser, 2020; Medpac, 2015).

Equitable allocation of resources is an ever-increasing challenge as technology improves and lives are extended through natural and mechanical means.

Resource allocation at the beginning and end of life is projected to continue to grow significantly! (Ford, 2015; Hartman et al., 2008).

All of these factors place greater stress on an already inefficient and overburdened healthcare system and results in more difficult ethical decisions about workforce allocation and equitable distribution of financial resources.

> **CLINICAL RELEVANCE**
>
> The principle of justice is of course integrated into the patient/client management role, but it is also heavily involved in the administration role of the physical therapist. For appropriate allocation of resources, Principles 7A, 7F, and 8B, and 8C of the Code of Ethics should be considered: **7A:** Physical therapists shall promote practice environments that support autonomous and accountable professional judgments. **7F:** Physical therapists shall refrain from employment arrangements, or other arrangements, that prevent physical therapists from fulfilling professional obligations to patients/clients. **8B:** Physical therapists shall advocate to reduce health disparities and healthcare inequities, improve access to healthcare services, and address the health, wellness, and preventive healthcare needs of people. **8C:** Physical therapists shall be responsible stewards of healthcare resources and shall avoid overutilization or underutilization of physical therapy services.

The Principle of Veracity

Veracity (truthfulness) is not a foundational bioethical principle and is granted just a passing mention in most ethics texts. It is at its core an element of respect for persons (Gabard and Martin, 2003). Veracity is antithetical to the concept of medical paternalism, which assumes patients need to know only what their physicians choose to reveal. Obviously there has been a dramatic change in attitudes toward veracity because it forms the basis for the autonomy expected by patients today. Informed consent, for example, is the ability to exercise autonomy with knowledge.

Decisions about withholding information involve a conflict between veracity and deception. There are times when the legal system and professional ethics agree that deception is legitimate and legal. **Therapeutic privilege** is invoked when the healthcare team makes the decision to withhold information believed to be detrimental to the patient. Such privilege is by its nature subject to challenge.

At times patients choose to not have the truth shared either with themselves or with their family, however, there is a basic belief that their healthcare provider is honest, truthful, and respectful and that personally and professionally the PT is truthful in all situations. We will address this again when we look at the expectations that society has for their PT and how the role of the PT is intertwined with the provider's personal life.

> **CLINICAL RELEVANCE**
>
> The principle of veracity is expected across all five roles of the physical therapist. Truthfulness is expected, and it is consistent with Principle 4A. **4A:** Physical therapists shall provide truthful, accurate, and relevant information and shall not make misleading representations.

The Principle of Fidelity

Fidelity is loyalty. It is not a foundational principle; however, we mention it here briefly as it speaks to the special relationship developed between patients and their PTs. Each owes the other loyalty; although the greater burden is on the medical provider, increasingly the patient must assume some of the responsibility (Beauchamp and Childress, 2001). Fidelity often results in a dilemma, because a commitment made to a patient may not result in the best outcome for that patient (Veatch, 2016). At the root of fidelity is the importance of keeping a promise, or of being true to your word. Individuals see this differently. Some are able to justify the importance of the promise at almost any cost, and others are able to set aside the promise if an action could be detrimental to the patient.

> **CLINICAL RELEVANCE**
>
> The concept of fidelity is the foundation of the patient/therapist relationship, and it is consistent with Principle 2A. **2A:** Physical therapists shall adhere to the core values of the profession and shall act in the best interests of patients/clients over the interests of the physical therapist.

THE MORAL THRESHOLD AND MORAL POTENCY

Each of us has a **moral threshold**, a bar below which we will not compromise. To compromise below your moral threshold is to compromise your personal integrity (Janoff-Bulman et al., 2009). Professional ethics raises that bar to a higher level. Professional ethics are only incumbent upon those who hold a specified role. There is an expectation that is associated with professionalism that recognizes the responsibility of the professional to act in a certain way, and that level of professional behavior is what is expected by the public and in exchange the public grants certain privileges to the professional. When a person chooses to enter a profession, they agree to take on the responsibilities associated with that professional role. It is often a topic of discussion as to why a healthcare provider is held to a higher standard and why the healthcare provider is expected to uphold that standard in their professional and public life. This is not optional; it is what is mandated by the social contract that is implicit in becoming a healthcare provider and entering into the patient/provider relationship. The central core of the social contract that forms the patient/provider relationship is trust.

A national study conducted in 2007 (Rosenthal et al., 2007) found that 77% of the participants either agreed or strongly agreed that there was a lack of confidence on America's leaders. The business literature has flourished recently, in the wake of many corporate scandals, and the findings are relevant to doing business in the not-for-profit healthcare environment as well (Welsh and Ordonez, 2014; Xu and Ma, 2016). Hannah and colleagues (2010) proposed that there is a key element missing from ethical leadership, which they refer to as *moral potency*. The basis of their work stems from the question: Why do leaders who know what is the right ethical decision, fail to take action, even when action is clearly necessary? (Schaubroeck et al., 2010).

Ethical behavior is not as strongly influenced by judgment as it is by *acting on* a moral judgment. Hannah and colleagues (2011a) define **moral potency** as "the capacity to generate responsibility, and motivation to take moral action in the face of adversity and to persevere through challenges."

Moral potency is built on (1) **moral ownership,** a sense of responsibility to take ethical action when faced with ethical issues; (2) **moral efficacy,** the beliefs of individuals that they can organize and mobilize to carry out an ethical action; and (3) **moral courage,** the courage to face threats and overcome fears to act (Goud, 2005; Hannah et al., 2009, 2011b; Morley et al., 2020).

PTs have become increasingly aware that the relationships that they develop with a patient must involve the ability to not only recognize an ethical challenge but also to act on that challenge independent of conflicting personal, institutional, or societal conflicts that may interfere with their judgment. Future chapters will provide very practical examples of the challenges inherent in situations that require moral potency.

THE RELATIONSHIP OF ETHICS AND THE LAW

There is an ongoing debate about the relationship of ethics and law. In 1958, the *Harvard Law Review* published the famous Hart Fuller Debate, which addressed the relationship of law and ethics (*Harvard Law Review*, 1958). Hart stated morality and law are separate, and Fuller opined that morality is the source of laws'

TABLE 1-1 ISSUES ADDRESSED BY BOTH ETHICS AND LAW

Access to medical care

Informed consent

Confidentiality

Exceptions to confidentiality

Mandatory reporting

Privileged communication with healthcare providers

Advance directives

Abortion

Physician-assisted suicide

binding power. Ethics and law both address similar issues (Table 1-1) and as licensed healthcare providers we have in addition to our professional ethical obligation the responsibility to know and adhere to the law. There are times that both legal and ethical adherence is required and other times that they do not both come into play in our actions simultaneously.

It has been said that the relationship of ethics and law considers that conscience is the guardian in the individual (ethics) for the rules which the community has evolved for its own preservation (law). There are limits to the law. The law cannot make people honest, caring, or fair. For example, lying, or betraying a confidence, is not illegal but it is unethical. While not every physical therapy practice act requires adherence to a code of ethics, all do require adherence to the law. What often baffles regulatory organizations whether based within an organization or ones that have government oversight is how to manage breaches of professional behavior that may or may not have also resulted in breaking a law but which are confounded by the individuals' apparent lack of understanding of their professional ethical responsibilities. These individuals have difficulty analyzing a future situation and determining that it will result in a breach of trust and will ultimately impact negatively on patient care. While they may have clinical skills that are judged competent, the equally important professional skills are lacking. The tools for good decision making are available, the laws governing the practice of physical therapy are specific to each jurisdiction, and it is the responsibility of each licensee to know the law and be able to apply it (www.fsbpt.org). Similarly, the APTA Code of Ethics for the Physical Therapist and the Standards of Ethical Conduct for the Physical Therapist Assistant guide the ethical behavior of all PT practitioners (www.apta.org).

CLINICAL RELEVANCE

While not every practice act addresses ethical issues directly, Principle 5A of the Code of Ethics very specifically addresses adherence to the law: **5A:** Physical therapists shall comply with applicable local, state, and federal laws and regulations. It is interesting to note that in research done regarding the reasons that people chose to sue healthcare providers for malpractice the number one reason is not necessarily as a result of an act of clinical negligence but more often because they feel there was a breach of the patient/practitioner relationship and in particular a breach in veracity.

Ideas to Consider

1. Ethical decision-making has become more complex because:
   a. The Hippocratic Oath has long been outdated.
   b. Society today is steeped in immorality.
   c. Organizational priorities and financial pressures affect everyday decisions.
   d. There are just so many more rules today than in earlier times.

2. At the center of the patient/therapist relationship is:
   a. Loyalty.
   b. Affection.
   c. Sincerity.
   d. Trust.

3. Healthcare ethics are unique because:
   a. Patients are vulnerable.
   b. A lot of money is involved.
   c. Healthcare workers care about people.
   d. Patients have complete autonomy.

4. An evolving standard of autonomy supports patients but must be balanced with:
   a. Demonstrated skills in ethical decision-making.
   b. A willingness to partner responsibly with their provider.
   c. Effective use of the Internet to gather facts about their care.
   d. Absence of mental or emotional issues.

5. Beneficence means:
   a. Being kind.
   b. Doing little harm.
   c. Ensuring services for all.
   d. Encouraging independence.

6. Nonmaleficence means:
   a. First of all, assess your patient.
   b. Not being malicious.
   c. Doing no harm.
   d. Avoiding malpractice.

7. Justice means:
   a. Fairness.
   b. Judgment.
   c. Sincerity.
   d. Legal.

8. Veracity means:
   a. Paternalism.
   b. Therapeutic privilege.
   c. Legitimacy.
   d. Truthfulness founded on a respect for persons.

9. When you lower your moral threshold, you:
   a. Compromise your integrity.
   b. Open your mind to new ideas.
   c. Increase your awareness of complex issues.
   d. Recognize the reality of healthcare.

10. Moral potency is:
    a. Repeating an action until you get the results you want.
    b. The capacity to take moral action responsibly in the face of adversity.
    c. Being willing to express your religious beliefs across all settings.
    d. Doing the right thing.

11. A hospital is about to break ground for a new wing. People chain themselves to a number of old trees that will be lost if the building goes forward. These people are behaving:
    a. Legally but unethically.
    b. Legally and ethically.
    c. Unethically and illegally.
    d. Ethically but illegally.

CHAPTER 2

The Evolution of the Code of Ethics for Physical Therapists and the Standards of Ethical Conduct of the Physical Therapist Assistant

There have been many attempts to provide a simple explanation or definition of the word profession and the individual who is a professional. The attempt always seems to center around an ethical foundation within an established expertise and established body of information. A profession has aptly been defined as a "disciplined group of individuals who adhere to ethical standards (Australian Council of Professions, 2022; Professional Standards Councils, 2022). A professional is an individual who identifies with a certain profession and adheres to the ethical standards of that group (Creuss et al., 2004).

A profession must have at its foundation a Code of Ethics that reflects the activities of the profession and the behaviors expected of the members of that profession. The Code of Ethics of a health care profession demands a higher standard of behavior in respect to the services provided to the public and the responsibility the health care provider has to the public and to professional colleagues (Bernard 2016; Evetts, 2011).

Having a distinct Code of Ethics is a mark of being a professional. Professionals bound by a Code of Ethics accept the right and obligations to accept the standards set, and to embrace the challenge of self-regulation of behavior and actions. Collectively the membership of an organization through its Code of Ethics upholds the profession's image and reputation.

The profession of physical therapy had its nascent beginnings in 1921 when a small group of women founded what would soon be called The American Physical Therapy Association, but it was not until 14 years later in 1935 that the first Code of Ethics and Discipline was adopted at the Physical Therapy Association's annual meeting in Atlantic City, New Jersey. The initial Code explicitly defined the responsibilities of the PT, but also drew a clear picture of behaviors expected of physical therapists. The Code provided direction at that time that later evolved over the years as the profession grew and developed. In 1935 the following specific guidance was provided for the practicing PT.

1. The physician's prescription has primacy in carrying out physical therapy treatments.
2. It is prohibited to procure patients through advertising.
3. Physical therapists cannot criticize physicians and colleagues in the presence of patients.

The Code of Ethics reflected the early practice patterns of the profession, PT was provided by referral only. Physical therapists practiced only under the direction of a physician with no practice autonomy or independent decision-making. It was another 13 years before the next revision of the Code of Ethics in 1948. Physical therapy had proven its importance during and following World War II, and soon after the war found itself at the epicenter of care during the polio epidemic that began in the early 1950s and spanned the first part of the decade. The 1948 revision of the Code of Ethics reflected little growth in professional autonomy on the part of the PTs. While still far from independent in their practice the profession of physical therapy was becoming more familiar to the public.

Significant components of the Code provided the following guidance to the PT practitioner.

1. The PT must have adequate medical supervision.
2. Diagnosis of disability and prescription of physical therapy is the responsibility of the physician only.
3. The PT is expected to give full support to the organization that the PT serves.
4. The PT is guided by the welfare of the patient.
5. The PT has the duty to disclose unethical activities of members and to testify in an investigation.

While PT practice was still very much under the purview of physician direction, and the PT was not encouraged to think independently in terms of their organization relationship, this revision of the Code of Ethics began to address some of the expected professional responsibility of the practicing clinician, for example, the PT is guided by the welfare of the patient, reinforcing the importance of the physical therapist/patient relationship. In addition, the professional responsibility of the therapist to protect patients through the privilege of self-regulation is first mentioned in this Code revision making it clear that the PT has an obligation to self-monitor with a duty to disclose unethical actions. This demonstrated to the public that the PT took their obligation to the public very seriously.

The Code of Ethics remained essentially unchanged for the next thirty years. In 1978 the Code was revised again. Health care delivery particularly payment changed significantly during that time. Employment-based insurance and Government entitlement programs like Medicare and Medicaid changed the payment landscape.

The Standards of Ethical Conduct for the Physical Therapist Assistant had also been developed. A Guide to Professional Conduct was added to the professional guidance documents for the PT to assist in interpreting the Code of Ethics. There were a few significant changes to the Code.

1. The Code encouraged sound judgment by the physical therapist.
2. PTs must conduct themselves as to not discredit the association and the profession.
3. Loyalty and support to the American Physical Therapy Association.
4. Reasonable and sound remuneration.
5. Written referral regardless of state law.

There were some interesting juxtapositions in this revision. While PTs are encouraged to take professional responsibility for their own actions, both in exhibiting sound judgment and conducting themselves as professionals, at the time of this revision only one jurisdiction permitted direct access to physical therapy services. However, the concept of direct access was very much on the agenda for physical therapy as a practice community. The Association, through the Code of Ethics took a position that regardless of what is legislated for patient access, physical therapists practicing legally through direct access would be considered to be practicing unethically. The Association has of course taken a much different approach over time, as direct access became one of the tenets of Vision 2020.

Over the next 30 years the Code of Ethics evolved, consistent with some of the changes in practice. In 2009 the Code of Ethics had 11 principles, the Standards of Ethical Conduct for the PTA which was adopted in the 1980's had seven principles. The following principles/standards were the same for the PT and the PTA:

1. Respect the rights and dignity/provide competent care.
2. Be trustworthy.
3. Comply with laws and regulations.
4. Professional competence for the PT and competence for the PTA.
5. Protect the public from unethical, illegal, incompetent acts.

The PT also had the following principles for guidance:

1. High standards: Practice/Research/Education.
2. Address the health needs of society.
3. Respect colleagues and other health care professionals.
4. Have sound professional judgment.
5. Reasonable remuneration.
6. Provide accurate and relevant information to the public.

The PTA had the following standards for guidance:

1. Supervision and direction of the PT.
2. Judgement commensurate with education and legal qualifications.

The APTA defined seven Core Values for the physical therapist. These were not incorporated in the Code of Ethics, however they were closely aligned with the expected behaviors of the PT and recently applied to the behaviors of the PTA as well:

Accountability
Altruism
Compassion/caring
Excellence
Integrity
Professional Duty
Social Responsibility
Collaboration was added later as it was recognized how important this value is to safe and effective patient care.

The Ethics and Judicial Committee of the APTA became quite concerned in the early part of the 21st century that physical therapists were practicing with critically important core documents that were over three decades old. At that time, The Ethics and Judicial Committee (EJC) of the APTA was charged annually to review both the Code of Ethics and the Guide for Professional Conduct and make recommendations to the House of Delegates regarding changes to the documents as necessary. In their work to adjudicate ethical issues that came before the committee, members were finding that the Code of Ethics was not robust enough to provide guidance about the many contemporary ethical issues impacting professional behavior. Beginning in 2005 the Ethics and Judicial Committee began a process to thoroughly evaluate the Code of Ethics, and the Standards of Ethical Conduct for the PTA for their relevance and applicability to contemporary practice. The Ethics and Judicial Committee embarked on an extensive review of the Code of Ethics for similar health care associations to inform the committee of best practices for similar organizations. Following this review, it was determined that the Ethics and Judicial Committee would provide the evidence and rationale for APTA to embark on an extensive review of the current Code of Ethics and Standards with recommendations for revisions as indicated. The primary question as the profession embraced Vision 2020 and the future of PT practice was, "Do the APTA core documents guide the autonomous practice of physical therapy as a doctoring profession?" The ethics and judicial committee determined that the current document was inadequate, at a minimum, the current document failed to address the following.

1. The role of the physical therapist as an educator, critical inquirer, Consultant and administrator was not addressed. The Code of Ethics had the narrow focus on the responsibilities of the physical therapist as a patient client manager only.
2. The Code of Ethics did not provide guidance about how to manage the responsibilities and demands of the PT related to autonomous/independent practice.
3. The Code did not address the complexities within the contemporary health care environment.

4. In addition, the Code and the Standards did not focus on the nuances of the relationship between the PT and the PTA and the relationship of both to other health care providers.

What was perhaps most disturbing was the Code of Ethics failed to articulate in any meaningful way the moral understanding that is unique to the profession of physical therapy. What is it about the patient-therapist relationship that requires an appreciation by the physical therapist and the physical therapist assistant of the privilege, and the inherent obligations associated with the PT patient therapeutic interaction?

The APTA Board of Directors agreed to the extensive review of the Code of Ethics and appointed a task force to undertake this significant undertaking. It was determined at the same time to look at the Standards for Ethical Conduct for the PTA to see if better alignment could be achieved between the two documents reflecting the collaborative and integrated nature of the practice of PT's and PTA's.

Revision of a document such as the Code of Ethics requires the input from multiple sources and extensive resources as it is the foundation of the moral fiber of the profession and all those who "profess" to be physical therapists. The revision of the Code of Ethics and the Standards of Ethical Conduct were completed in parallel as it was critical that the documents were in concert with each other, and complemented one another. A task force consisting of thirteen physical therapists (including four EJC members), one physical therapist assistant, one student and one physical therapy regulator was appointed by the Board to formulate and initiate the process. The entire process took place over almost four years from inception to completion to enactment in 2010, The new documents reflected the current practice environment but also projected where practice was anticipated to go in the next few years. The new Code was consistent with the APTA vision statement at the time that envisioned a doctoring profession with patients having direct access to PT services. In 2022, the APTA Board of Directors appointed a new task force to review the Code and Standards and make recommendations to the Board regarding the currency and applicability of both to the current practice of physical therapy.

A Code of Ethics has to be a dynamic document, based on universal principles and values that demonstrate professional duties and expectations. The Code must provide guidance that is meaningful and applied to the realities of physical therapy practice. The Code has to be assimilated into professional practice and recognized as the core foundational document for ethical behavior by those that will use it. Ethical decision making is a learned skill, and the application of the Code requires meaningful opportunities to apply the principles and concepts.

The current Code of Ethics fundamentally has a very different design than the documents that preceded it. Addressing the limitations of the prior documents the current code of ethics begins with a preamble identifying the contemporary roles of the physical therapist and the "special obligation of the physical therapist to empower, educate, and enable those with impairments, activity limitations, participation restrictions, and disabilities to facilitate greater independence, health, wellness and enhanced quality of life." The format is meant to be inclusive with the lettered principles expanding upon the numbered principles that clarify intent, meaning and application. All principles begin with the common phrase of "physical therapists shall" raising every principle to the level of an ethical obligation. The core values of the physical therapy profession are incorporated into the code and associated with each group of principles. The preamble further delineates the ethical obligation of all physical therapists as defined by the American Physical Therapy Association. The preamble also makes the purpose of the Code of Ethics clear to all physical therapists and physical therapy students who are bound by the code as well as patients and other stakeholders who interact with physical therapists. The purposes of the Code are the following:

1. Provide standards of behavior and performance that form the basis of professional accountability to the public.
2. Provide guidance for physical therapists facing ethical challenges.
3. Educate physical therapists, students, other health care professionals, regulators and the public regarding the ethical obligations of the physical therapist.
4. Establish the standards by which the American Physical Therapy Association can determine if a physical therapist has engaged in unethical conduct.

The Code and Standards provided clarification for long-standing ethical obligations that were part of the original code and each subsequent revision. Ethical obligations toward patients and colleagues, the duty of respect the virtues of truthfulness, honesty, and integrity. The revised documents, recognizing the complexities of contemporary practice go beyond the original code, providing guidance in the individual, Organizational and societal realms.

While elements of the original documents have carried over into the current code, there is new guidance that reflects what the physical therapy community identified as issues of ethical concern at the time the Code was being revised. This included the obligation to take personal responsibility for professional competence through lifelong engagement with the profession. The importance of encouraging, cultivating and developing best practices for service delivery and discouraging business practices that are not in the patient's best interest and finally the critical need to address the social determinants of health in impact our society and help to make physical therapy services accessible.

The last three principles are very important additions to the Code of Ethics and Standards, but they will not be the last. Some changes have been made to the Code of Ethics since first adopted in 2010, clarifying language and adding the important virtue of collaboration, as a core value, that speaks to our obligation to work with others within our discipline as well as other disciplines to provide the best care possible. Future issues that may need ethical guidance remain to be seen, but like any profession as we mature the complexities of our profession will continue to evolve new ethical issues. We already know that social inequity, respect for our environment and our natural resources, social media challenges, the impact of unethical behavior on patients and the profession are challenges that confront everyone in health care and how they are resolved will define much of how the profession of physical therapy grows in the future. We also recognize that as we continue to grow

Principle/Standard	Ethical Guidance	Added in 2010
1	Duty to all individuals	
2	Duty to patients/clients	
3	Accountability for sound judgment	
4	Integrity in relationships	
5	Fulfilling legal and professional obligations	
6	Lifelong acquisition of knowledge, skills, abilities	X
7	Organizational behavior and business practices	X
8	Meeting the health needs of society	X

as a profession and become more comfortable in our professional evolution every clinician has to be empowered to own their professional behavior and take responsibility for individual and organizational professional growth.

Ideas to Consider

1. What type of document is a professional Code of Ethics?
   a. Static.
   b. Dynamic.
   c. Transient.
   d. All of the above.

2. Which statement is true about health care professions?
   a. All have a guidance document like a Code of Ethics.
   b. Most have a guidance document like a Code of Ethics.
   c. Some have a guidance document like a Code of Ethics.
   d. Only hands-on health care fields have a Code of Ethics.

3. Which statement is true about the current Code of ethics and standards of ethical conduct?
   a. The Code and Standards belong to the APTA.
   b. The Code and Standards are binding on all PTs and PTAs not just APTA members.
   c. The numbered and lettered principles and standards are equally important.
   d. All the above are true.

CHAPTER 3

Professionalism

Physical therapy in the United States evolved from its technical roots in the early 20th century to its current level of development, it is expected that a critical mass of practicing clinicians will have a Doctor of Physical Therapy degree by 2025 (APTA, 2014). The demands on the physical therapist to collaborate and practice as part of the inter-professional team continue to grow requiring further development and refinement of clinical skills. These clinical skills include the skills in ethical decision making that we will concentrate on in this text.

The roots of physical therapy go all the way back to 400 BC when Hippocrates and Galen advocated for treatment that included massage, manual therapy, and hydrotherapy. In the 18th century, orthopedists employed exercise as part of their treatment. In 1813, the Royal Central Institute of Gymnastics was founded in Sweden and therapeutic exercise became part of medical practice. In 1887, Sweden started registering practitioners of "physiotherapy." In 1894, four nurses founded the Chartered Society of Physiotherapists. In 1913, the New Zealand School of Physiotherapy was founded, and in 1914, the first cohort of Reconstruction Aides, the precursors to physical therapists graduated from Reed College in the United States. In December 1921 several visionary women met in New York City recognizing the importance of establishing the nascent profession of physical therapy in the United States. This group of leaders established the 238-member strong, "American Women's Physical Therapeutic Association." A year later, in the first effort to be inclusive, not excluding their male colleague, the organization changed the name to the American Physiotherapy Association.

Physical therapy grew rapidly as a result of two world wars, and Polio, a major pandemic. Both events threatened the lives of many, yet lives were spared with the help of major medical advancements, including the development of antibiotics, safer blood transfusions, improvements in infection control, and surgical innovations, which saved people on the battlefield, and at home, leaving them alive but with disabilities to conquer. Medicine further evolved through the 1950's, though still physician-centric during that period, physical therapy continued to evolve.

In the 1960s, the culture was to question and distrust authority, and medicine was not immune to that mentality, resulting in the further development of ancillary services and alternative healthcare treatments. People began to take more responsibility for their own healthcare needs. The relationship of provider and patient/client continues to evolve as information available to individuals to manage their own healthcare continues to grow in quantity and availability.

While physical therapy started as a technical field it has evolved into a profession. The Australian Council of Professions defines a profession as a, "disciplined group of individuals who adhere to ethical standards and who hold themselves out as, and are accepted by the public as possessing special knowledge and skills in a widely recognized body of learning derived from research, education, and training at a high level, and who are prepared to apply this knowledge and exercise these skills in the interest of others." (Australian Council, 2023)

A member of a profession is a professional, and consistent with the social contract between the PT profession and the public, it is expected that the professional will behave ethically with the virtues among others of integrity, trust, and expertise (Queensland Nurse 2011, Starr, 2023).

Society trusts healthcare professionals to uphold the core values that are the foundation of the profession, and the professional agrees to maintain the patient as the central focus of the healthcare system. The ability to self-regulate is grated to healthcare providers because of the inherent trust that the healthcare providers' interests are altruistic and in the best interest of the patient/client (Figure 3-1).

The patient–therapist relationship is based on three pillars. First, trust is required of both the PT and the patient. Integrity, one of the core values, is another foundational principle and is the bedrock that secures the trust the patient has in the therapist. The final pillar is legitimacy, which is recognized as the practitioner demonstrating initial competence and consistently maintaining the knowledge base throughout their professional career. It is also dependent on effectiveness, increasingly more important all the time as we carefully manage our resources, so we keep the principle of justice in the forefront and manage to provide services to as many as possible safely and effectively (Starr, 2019).

As has been noted previously, Society has certain expectations of professionals, and in return for the fulfillment of those expectations, Society willingly gives professions (and their professionals) certain privileges (Table 3-1).

The physical therapist must be cognizant that while they have chosen a healthcare field with demanding professional responsibilities, there must be a balance with personal obligations so a healthy life balance can be maintained. There are many suggestions on how to accomplish this and all of them include recommendations that involve competence and ethical behavior. The competent physical therapist who is comfortable with their clinical skill ability and their ethical decision-making feels comfortable as a practitioner. Some of the suggestions for maintaining this critical Personal Professional Life balance are shown in Table 3-2.

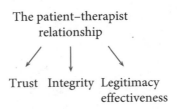

Figure 3-1 Pillars of the patient–therapist relationship.

TABLE 3-1 SOCIETAL EXPECTATIONS

Society's Expectations of Us	Our Expectations of Society
• Healing • Patient-focussed • Competent • Altruistic • Integrity/morality • Promotion of public good • Accountability • Lifelong learner	• Monopoly • Autonomy • Input into public policy • Status financial reward • Respect • Self-regulation

Source: Data from Cruess (2006) and updated by Price (2015).

TABLE 3-2 PERSONAL AND PROFESSIONAL LIFE BALANCE

Life Balance Recommendation	Rationale
Lifelong commitment to learning	Stay current to stay competent
Ethical behavior at all times	Ethical decisions on behalf of our patients are constant
Manage your finances with an eye to your future	Financial security helps to clear the way to making choices without a conflict of interest
Manage your time	Recognize what you can and cannot do in a given amount of time
Set your priorities	Family matters ... Patients matter, set your priorities as circumstances permit
Develop your expertise	Allow your passion to help establish and cultivate your expertise
Look below and above your generation	Seek the advice of those with more experience and the energy of those that follow you
Go beyond what is expected	Always strive to exceed patients' and colleagues' expectations
Don't procrastinate	Unmet deadlines are stressful, while a necessary part of life it should not have a negative impact on productivity

Source: Adapted from Baum (2008).

Healthcare professionalism has become a field of study on its own because the effective delivery of healthcare services does not rely on just clinical skills. Professional behavior is a very large aspect of effective healthcare, yet they are skills that are much more difficult to teach, and students will clearly indicate that the "softer" professional skills are not as highly valued by students. Unfortunately, these critical skills have been inappropriately named over the years. They are not "soft skills" rather they are survival skills. Research in the area of delivering healthcare services most effectively has centered on the principles that are described in the C.L.E.A.R. protocol (Sullivan, Luallin Group, 2017), but similar protocols have been adopted by other institutions. The protocol suggests that the healthcare provider *connects*, *listens*, *explains*, *asks*, and *reconnects*. An important note here is that while we have access to technology that enhances our practice capability, we have to be very cognizant that anything that could be perceived as a communication barrier will disrupt the patient–therapist relationship. So, a tablet/laptop is a tremendous asset, but we have to make sure it does not become a barrier to communication. Professionalism is the mark of being a professional and the trust that is the core of the clinician-patient relationship is critical.

Ideas to Consider

1. The patient–therapist relationship is based on:
   a. Integrity.
   b. Trust.
   c. Legitimacy.
   d. Effectiveness.
   e. (a) & (b).
   f. All of the above.

2. Legitimacy is linked to:
   a. Integrity.
   b. Competence.
   c. Altruism.
   d. Relevance.

3. Professional skills are best named:
   a. Structural skills.
   b. Survival skills.
   c. Soft skills.
   d. Hard skills.

CHAPTER 4

Ethical Guidance: The Code of Ethics for Physical Therapists and Standards of Ethical Conduct for the Physical Therapist Assistant

Ethical guidance is not static. Ethical demands on therapists have changed as practice demands have changed. With direct access in all fifty jurisdictions and the District of Columbia, the Code of Ethics was reviewed for its applicability to today's more complicated practice demands. It was determined that the Code of Ethics no longer provided adequate guidance to practitioners facing more ethical issues as a result of more independent practice. A complete revision was adopted by the House of Delegates of the American Physical Therapy Association (APTA) and it went into effect on July 1, 2010 (Kirsch, 2009). A new task force was named in 2022 and will be making recommendations about the Code and the Standards in 2023.

To best understand and appreciate the differences between the current and old documents, it is important to compare and contrast the documents, particularly the preamble. The preamble sets "the stage" for the difference between the old documents and the current documents.

The old preambles simply state that physical therapists (PTs) are responsible for promoting ethical practice and that physical therapist assistants (PTAs) are responsible for maintaining high standards of conduct while acting in the best interests of patients/clients.

The preamble to the current Code* establishes the uniqueness of physical therapy as a profession—emphasizing that, as PTs perform multiple roles across a variety of settings, the ethical principles and standards of conduct with which they are expected to comply apply regardless of role or venue. A foundation of autonomy,

---

*The Code of Ethics and Standards of Ethical Conduct are available at: http:// www.apta.org/Ethics Professionalism/

responsibility, and accountability is established in the preamble and resonates through the Code.

The preamble to the current Standards of Ethical Conduct, meanwhile, cites the PTA's obligation to facilitate patients'/clients' achievement of greater independence, health, and wellness.

Both current preambles note that the documents are not exhaustive and do not address every situation. The Code and Standards provide guidance and consultation with colleagues using the Code and standards is the best way to manage ethical problems. The Code of Ethics for the physical therapist and the standards of Ethical Conduct for the physical therapist assistant are documents that belong to the American Physical Therapy Association, the professional association. They are binding on all PTs and PTAs regardless of whether they are Association members.

THE PRINCIPLES AND STANDARDS

The principles enumerated in the Code build on core values of accountability, altruism, compassion, excellence, integrity, professional duty, collaboration and social responsibility. These values are described in the APTA document Professionalism in Physical Therapy: Core Values (available at "Core Documents").

Both the principles of the Code and the standards of the Standards of Ethical Conduct reflect the uniqueness of the field of physical therapy (APTA, 2017a; 2017b). Both documents establish for practitioners, employers, employees, and, most importantly, the public the responsibility that PTs and PTAs assume for their own and their colleagues' ethi- cal behavior. Both documents also reflect the challenges and opportunities presented by the various practice environments in which physical therapy services are provided.

This chapter will provide a brief introduction for each Principle and Standard.

Principle 1/Standard 1

Principle 1 and Standard 1 illustrate the duty of PTs and PTAs, respectively, to serve all people. Principle 1 reflects the core values of compassion, caring and integrity.

Principle 1 and Standard 1 offer considerable guidance. Both state that PTs/PTAs "shall respect the inherent dignity and rights of all individuals" and "shall act in a respectful manner toward each person regardless of age, gender, race, nationality, religion, ethnicity, social or economic status, sexual orientation, health condition or disability." Principle 1 states that PTs shall "recognize personal biases and shall not discriminate against others in physical therapist practice, consultation, education, research, and administration." Similarly, Standard 1 states that PTAs shall "recognize personal biases and shall not discriminate against others in the provision of physical therapy services."

The take-home message of Principle 1 and Standard 1 is that PTs and PTAs respect each patient or client without bias, recognizing their own personal biases and doing their best to prevent those biases from affecting patient/client care.

Principle 2/Standard 2

Principle 2 and Standard 2 illustrate the obligation of PTs and PTAs to meet the needs of their patients. Principle 2 reflects the core values of altruism, collaboration, compassion, caring and professional duty.

The documents go into much greater detail. Both Principle 2 and Standard 2 state that PTs/PTAs shall be "trustworthy and compassionate in addressing the rights and needs of patients/clients," act "in the best interests of patients/clients" rather than in the best interests of the PT/PTA, provide "services" (Principle 2) or "physical therapy interventions" (Standard 2) with "compassionate and caring behaviors that incorporate the individual and cultural differences of patients/clients," and "protect confidential patient/client information."

Principle 2 further directs PTs to "provide the information necessary to allow patients or their surrogates to make informed decisions about physical therapy care or participation in clinical research"; Standard 2 directs PTAs to "provide patients/clients with information regarding the interventions they provide."

Principle 2 states it is the duty of PTs to "collaborate with patients/clients to empower them in decisions about their health care" and that PTs may disclose confidential patient/client information to appropriate authorities "only when allowed or as required by law. "

The take-home message here is that PTs and PTAs respect patients' and clients' autonomy by giving them the information they need to make informed decisions. Furthermore, the PT helps patients and clients with their decision making, and both the PT and PTA—the latter in collaboration with the PT—protect the patient's or client's confidentiality.

Principle 3/Standard 3

Principle 3 and Standard 3 emphasize the need for PTs and PTAs to exercise sound judgment based on objectivity and informed decision making. Collaboration, Duty, Excellence and integrity are the highlighted core values in Principle 3.

Principle 3 specifies that PTs shall:

- Be accountable for making sound professional judgments;
- Demonstrate independent and objective professional judgment in the patient's/client's best interest in all practice settings;
- Demonstrate professional judgment informed by professional standards, evidence (including literature and established best practice), practitioner experience, and patient/client values; and
- Make judgments within their scope of practice and level of expertise; and communicate with, collaborate with, or refer to peers or other health professionals when necessary.

Similarly, Standard 3 adds considerable detail and direction specifying that PTAs shall:

- Make sound decisions in collaboration with the physical therapist and within the boundaries established by laws and regulations;
- Make objective decisions in the patient's/client's best interest in all practice settings;
- Be guided by information about best practice regarding physical therapy interventions;
- Make decisions based upon their level of competence and consistent with patient/client values;
- Not engage in conflicts of interest; and
- Provide physical therapy services under the direction and supervision of a physical therapist and communicate with the physical therapist when patient/client status requires modifications to the established plan of care.

The take-home message for PTs is that they exercise autonomous professional judgment, based on evidence and in collaboration with other healthcare professionals as necessary. For PTAs, the message is that they, working in collaboration with PTs, must make decisions that are in patients' and clients' best interest.

Principle 4/Standard 4

Principle 4 and Standard 4 call upon PTs and PTAs to demonstrate integrity in their relationships with patients/clients and others. What Principle 4 and Standard 4 do is spell out expected behaviors and actions related to such areas as exploitation, misconduct, suspected abuse, improper relationships, and harassment. Specifically, both Principle 4 and Standard 4 state that PTs/PTAs shall:

- Demonstrate integrity in their relationships with patients/clients, families, colleagues, students, other healthcare providers, employers, payers, and the public (for PTs, the obligation extends to research participants)—providing truthful, accurate, and relevant information, and not making misleading representations;
- Not exploit persons over whom they have supervisory, evaluative, or other authority (e.g., patients/clients, students, subordinates, research participants, or employees);
- Discourage misconduct by healthcare professionals and report illegal or unethical acts to the relevant authority, when appropriate;
- Report suspected cases of abuse involving children or vulnerable adults to [for PTAs, the supervising physical therapist and] the appropriate authority, subject to law;
- Not engage in any sexual relationship with any of their patients/clients, subordinates, or students; and
- Not harass anyone verbally, physically, emotionally, or sexually.

The take-home message is that PTs and PTAs are expected to act with integrity in relationships with patients, coworkers, students, and any other vulnerable individuals. Both PTs and PTAs are responsible for protecting vulnerable populations from harmful or potentially harmful behaviors.

Principle 5/Standard 5

Principle 5 and Standard 5 focus on legal and professional obligations. Principle 5 reflects the core values of professional duty and accountability, social responsibility.
Both Principle 5 and Standard 5 state that PTs/PTAs shall:

- Fulfill their legal and professional (for PTs) or ethical (for PTAs) obligations;
- Comply with applicable local, state, and federal laws and regulations;
- When involved in research, abide by accepted standards protection of research participants;
- Encourage to seek assistance or counsel colleagues with physical, psychological, or substance-related impairments that may adversely affect their professional responsibilities; and
- Report to the appropriate authority knowledge that a colleague is unable to perform his or her responsibilities with reasonable skill and safety.

Principle 5 also states that PTs "have primary responsibility for supervision of physical therapist assistants and support personnel," and dictates that they "provide notice and information about alternatives for obtaining care in the event the physical therapist terminates the provider relationship while the patient/client continues to need physical therapy services."

Standard 5 also states that PTAs "support the supervisory role of the physical therapist to ensure quality of care and promote patient/client safety."

The take-home message is that PTs and PTAs recognize that their legal and professional or ethical responsibilities may extend beyond what is required by practice acts and into the moral realm to protect patients, colleagues, and society.

Principle 6/Standard 6

Principle 6 and Standard 6 pertain to PTs' and PTAs' lifelong acquisition of knowledge and skills. Principle 6 reflects the core value of excellence.

Furthermore, PTs and PTAs are expected to "enhance their expertise [PTs]/competence [PTAs] through the lifelong acquisition and refinement of knowledge, skills, and abilities." Principle 6 for PTs adds "professional behaviors" to that list. PTs and PTAs likewise are directed to achieve and maintain competence "professional" competence in the case of PTs, "clinical" competence in the case of PTAs.

Principle 6 further states that PTs shall:

- Take responsibility for their professional development based on critical self-assessment and reflection on changes in physical therapist practice, education, health care delivery, and technology.
- Evaluate the strength of evidence and applicability of content presented during professional development activities before integrating the content or techniques into practice; and
- Cultivate practice environments that support professional development, lifelong learning, and excellence.

Standard 6 further directs PTAs to "engage in life-long learning consistent with changes in their roles and responsibilities and advances in the practice of physical therapy," and to "support practice environments that support career development and life-long learning."

The take-home message is that PTs and PTAs must stay current in enhancing their knowledge and skills. Furthermore, PTs must support patient care with evidence-based interventions.

Principle 7/Standard 7

Principle 7 and Standard 7 are related to organizational behaviors and business practices. Principle 7 reflects the core values of integrity and accountability.

Principle 7 states that PTs shall:

- Promote organizational behaviors and business practices that benefit patient/ clients and society;
- Promote practice environments that support autonomous and accountable professional judgments;
- Seek remuneration as is deserved and reasonable;
- Not accept gifts or other considerations that influence or give an appearance of influencing their professional judgment;
- Fully disclose any financial interest they have in products or services that they recommend to patients/clients;
- Be aware of charges and ensure that documentation and coding for physical therapy services accurately reflect the nature and extent of services provided; and
- Refrain from employment arrangements, or other arrangements, that prevent physical therapists from fulfilling professional obligations to patients/clients.

Standard 7 states that PTAs shall:

- Support organizational behaviors and business practices that benefit patients/ clients and society;
- Promote work environments that support ethical and accountable decision-making;
- Not accept gifts or other considerations that influence or give an appearance of influencing decisions;
- Fully disclose any financial interest they have in products or services that they recommend to patients/clients;
- Ensure that documentation for their interventions accurately reflects the nature and extent of the services provided; and
- Refrain from employment arrangements, or other arrangements, that prevent physical therapist assistants from fulfilling ethical obligations to patients/clients.

The take-home message is that PTs and PTAs accept responsibility for their actions, support full disclosure, and avoid employment relationships that prevent them from fulfilling their responsibilities to patients.

Principle 8/Standard 8

Principle 8 and Standard 8 pertain to meeting society's health needs. Principle 8 reflects the core value of social responsibility.

Both Principle 8 and Standard 8 state that PTs/PTAs "shall participate in efforts to meet the health needs of people locally, nationally, or globally."

Principle 8 adds that PTs shall:

- Provide pro bono physical therapy services or support organizations that meet the health needs of people who are economically disadvantaged, uninsured, and underinsured;
- Advocate to reduce health disparities and health care inequities, improve access to health care services, and address the health, wellness, and preventive health care needs of people;
- Be responsible stewards of health care resources and avoid overutilization or underutilization of physical therapy services; and
- Educate members of the public about the benefits of physical therapy and the unique role of the physical therapist.

Standard 8 adds that PTAs shall:

- Support organizations that meet the health needs of people who are economically disadvantaged, uninsured, and underinsured;
- Advocate for people with impairments, activity limitations, participation restrictions, and disabilities in order to promote their participation in the community and society;
- Be responsible stewards of health care resources by collaborating with physical therapists in order to avoid overutilization of physical therapy services; and
- Educate members of the public about the benefits of physical therapy.

The take-home message here is that PTs and PTAs help provide services to people whose access to physical therapy is limited. PTs and PTAs also acccept the responsibility to use services responsibly and help people understand the benefits of physical therapy.

SPANNING THE REALMS

The documents span the three realms of ethical action—individual, organizational, and societal—and devote considerable attention to challenging contemporary issues such as advocacy, organizational behavior, and business practices.

The Code and the Standards do not address every possible ethical situation, but the guidance they offer provides context for ethical decision making and the framework for addressing the ethical issues that confront therapists in all practice situations.

OWNING YOUR OWN PRACTICE

It is important to note that the Code of Ethics provides clear guidance to the physical therapist that they must embrace the idea that they have the responsibility to "own" every aspect of their own practice, meaning that they will be accountable for every action that they take. The principles of the Code of Ethics that strongly support the idea of accountability are as follows.

- **Principle 3**: PTs shall be accountable for making sound professional judgments.
- **Principle 6**: PTs shall enhance their expertise through the lifelong acquisition and refinement of knowledge, skills, abilities and professional behaviors.
- **Principle 7**: PTs shall promote organizational behaviors and business practices that benefit patients and clients and society.
    7A: Promote practice environments that support autonomous and accountable professional judgment.
- **Principle 8D**: PTs shall educate members of the public about the benefits of physical therapy and the unique role of the physical therapist.

Ideas to Consider

1. Why was a new Code of Ethics necessary?
   a. It was required by law.
   b. PTs are facing more ethical situations.
   c. We have a new Code of Ethics every 10 years.
   d. Other professions had new documents.

2. What does The Standard of Ethical Conduct provide?
   a. Explanation for the Code of Ethics.
   b. Guidance for the physical therapist.
   c. Guidance for the physical therapist assistant.
   d. Standards for PT administration.

3. Who is responsible to practice according to the Code of Ethics?
   a. All physical therapists.
   b. All physical therapist assistants.
   c. Only APTA members.
   d. (a) & (b)

4. The idea that every PT must "own their practice" means?
   a. PTs should only be in private practice.
   b. PTs must put money in their practice.
   c. PTs must be able to hire and fire people.
   d. Every PT must take responsibility for all aspects of their own practice.

CHAPTER 5

Ethical Risk Factors and Moral Injury

Knowing the right thing to do, doesn't always mean we will do it.

Healthcare professionals accept the obligation to answer to a set of ethical standards that are more demanding that those incumbent on the general population. Nobody expects that their ethical values will be challenged during their professional career, so the question arises why do people find themselves with ethical breaches and is there something they could have done to prevent these lapses? There has been little formal work done in this area. Some early observations and data, gathered primarily through interviewing individuals to see where moral breakdown may have occurred, resulted in some interesting findings. Across healthcare fields, medicine, nursing, and of course physical therapy, some common factors have been identified as not the only cause for an ethical breach but was certainly a contributing factor. Recognizing some of the potential contributing factors can be helpful for all practitioners in their effort to avoid an ethical behavioral lapse (Welsh and Ordonez, 2014).

Some of the most common factors are identified in Table 5-1. They are not in order of importance, as that depth of inquiry has not been done yet on ethical risk factors. The PT Professional Liability Exposure Claim Report from HPSO (CNA, 2020) identified many of the same risk factors for malpractice as have been identi-fied for ethical issues. The relationship of course is the expectation of professional behavior that lowers both ethical and liability risk.

TABLE 5-1 COMMON FACTORS RELATED TO ETHICAL BREACHES IN CONDUCT
Personal well-being
Non-US PT education
Power gradient pressure
Professional experience
Age
Professional isolation
Situational risk factors

It is helpful to explore each of these factors in a little more depth as they can serve as benchmarks for each of us to use as guideposts to determine our personal ethical risk level.

Personal well-being: One of the most important but most difficult things to do is a self-assessment to determine if our own personal physical and mental health is strong enough to manage the health and well-being of another person. This relates to having clearness of thought, so decision-making is based on logical thought processes using professional standards.

Non-US entry-level PT education: While the physical therapy education is substantially equivalent, the differences between healthcare delivery in the complicated US system and other nations make it more complicated to deliver care if the practitioner is not familiar with the healthcare system. The other situation that results in ethical breaches results from VISA concerns, where the PT may find themselves in circumstances where they are asked to do certain things that they consider doing out of fear of losing the job that is tied to their VISA.

Power gradient pressure: Physical therapists generally did not choose PT as a career because they wanted to be "in power," yet that is often the position PTs find themselves in, whether it is with patients whose position is one of vulnerability, or with students, employees, or research subjects. Ethical breaches are not uncommon on both sides of the power gradient, the person who is intimidated by the power and the one who is wielding the power. The other issue is the dual relationship that may result in uncomfortable situations as a result of the dual agency that exists when there is a therapeutic relationship and another one of equal value such as a personal relationship. These situations can be managed, but they must be recognized. For example, you may be the most competent practitioner with a certain skill set that would make you the logical choice to treat a close friend of yours. If you could refer them to a colleague, that would be preferable but not always possible.

Professional experience: There are two aspects of professional experience that must be considered. The first and most reasonable is a new graduate has had limited opportunity to experience a variety of situations. If they do not have good mentorship and guidance available to them, they will have little to rely on for ethical decision-making and could easily be misguided. The other aspect that must be considered is that any therapist regardless of experience when there is a change in practice setting even a very experienced therapist will confront situations that are unique to that setting, and they may have not have the professional expertise to manage those situations without guidance and mentorship.

Age: Age is of itself in a unique category as one would suspect that it should be related to experience, but it is not. Vulnerability for ethical and liability risk increases after age 45. The exact reason why this occurs is not known, but there is some conjecture that it has to do with becoming somewhat complacent and not seeing the input of others, which is most important in the process of ethical decision-making regardless of years or type of experience.

Professional isolation: The professional endeavor that we are involved in, healthcare is one that benefits from collaboration for both clinical decision-making as well as ethical decision-making. Professional education emphasizes this professional collaboration, so entry-level practitioners are comfortable with the group process that is beneficial to collaborative practice. There is greater recognition of the importance of interprofessional collaboration. Interprofessional practice has long been the norm in the rehabilitation world, but not as common in other areas of medicine. Often, collaboration is what students experience throughout their professional education but they do not see much evidence of interprofessional practice. In their work setting, they may find themselves less than engaged on a day-to-day basis with colleagues and lose sight of the importance of professional engagement. A solo practitioner can be very engaged professionally connecting with colleagues through the professional association and other professional activities. In contrast, a practitioner working with many colleagues can be professionally isolated by not engaging in professional discourse.

Situational risk factors: There are factors that when they occur in another circumstance may not be a problem. These may include work setting and power gradient issues. For example, an employee with little experience is asked to prepare a bill in a manner that they believe is incorrect. They raise their concern with their boss who makes it clear that they either follow the agency policy or seek employment elsewhere. A similar incident with a less vulnerable therapist could have a very different outcome.

There are other risk factors, but these are the most common. It is up to each of us to determine for ourselves what may be diverting our attention from fulfilling our patient-therapist obligation. Recognizing what some of these factors may be is important in keeping our professional focus. Establishing a professional network of trusted colleagues for clinical and professional consultation is critical in helping to maintain and promote professional balance.

Burnout or Moral Injury: The ethical ramifications:

Recently it has been noted that there is attrition from health care as a result of what is commonly referred to as burnout. While we might argue that burnout is not really the true reason for qualified clinicians to leave their profession, we do know that dissatisfaction with the professional role is a significant risk factor for clinicians and patients. If a clinician is unable to perform their responsibilities because of a physical or mental health reason, and they do not manage it effectively themselves the Code of Ethics and the Standards of Ethical Conduct are quite clear on the responsibility we have to monitor one another. **Principle 5E, Standard 5E**

PT's and PTA's who have knowledge that a colleague is unable to perform their professional responsibilities with reasonable skill and safety shall report this information to the appropriate authority.

The nature of work is quite different for the health care provider because of the responsibility and human interaction that occurs. Services are delivered to an individual but there is a societal impact as well. The provider has passion for the service delivered.

The services demand high quality all the time. It requires the use of cognitive and psychomotor skills simultaneously and considerable problem-solving and satisfaction seeking is occurring (Pruthi, 2019).

The average person spends 1/3 of their life at work. 90,000 hours

Health care providers spend more than 1/3 of their life at work ... and often work when "not at work" 111,571 hours. Physical therapy clinicians are passionate about the work they are privileged to be able to do. There is significant frustration when the ability to engage in their work is impacted negatively by the demands of the provision of care. Some of these demands are:

- Excessive paperwork
- Productivity demands
- Declining remuneration
- Decreased independence
- Government and payor demands
- Constant change
- Uncertainty.

(Dean et al., 2019)

When health care providers become frustrated with their inability to do their job as they would like to be able to do it there is a negative impact on the provision of care with an impact on patients, providers, the health care system.

- Patients
    - Harm related to provider error
    - Loss of trust
- Providers
    - Turnover
    - Substance abuse/Mental health
    - Suicide
- The Health Care System
    - Cost
    - Growth.

(Shanafelt, 2012; Archives Intern Med., 2012)

These are all of considerable concern as they have a significant impact on patient care. This is described as occupational burnout. Burnout is a multidimensional syndrome first described by Maslach, 1996, the signs of burnout are: Emotional/Physical exhaustion, Depersonalization, Reduced personal accomplishment, and Feelings of ineffectiveness. Burnout is considered to be an individual situation related to personal feelings of dissatisfaction. Burnout might not be accurately describing what is actually happening with PTs and PTAs. A more accurate description might be what was described by Shay in 1998 as **Moral Injury** (Shay 2014). Moral injury was initially associated with the military. Moral injury occurs when health care providers who are in high stakes situations feel that they cannot provide the standard of care that they and society demand of them, and the limitation is not from themselves but rather from a systemic failure.

Moral injury occurs when the clinician has Exposure to Potentially Morally Injurious Events (PMIE), PMIE's occur in high-stakes environments. They violate

TABLE 5-2 TERMINOLOGY ASSOCIATED WITH MORAL INJURY

Angry	Incompetent
Confused	Isolation
Conflicted	Lack of focus
Despair	Loss of trust
Disppointment	Remorse
Frustrated	Shame
Grief	Systemic failure
Guilt	Wronged
Helpless	

one's moral code or values (Borges et al., 2020). Moral injury can only be alleviated when obligations that conflict with the patient clinician relationship of trust are reduced, eliminated, or made to no longer be in conflict (Table 5-2). This requires some fundamental system changes (Pruthi, 2019).

The loss of competent health care workers as a result of burnout is a significant problem and addressing clinician burnout has been added as the fourth aim to the triple aim of controlling cost, improving the patient experience and improving population health (Maxim, 2022). The cost of moral injury is illustrated in Figure 5-1

To address how the systemic cause of moral injury can be addressed we need to have a better understanding of the root cause of moral injury.

- Lack of resilience
- Adaptability to cope
- Unrealistic expectations
- The health care system
  - Workload, time pressure, role ambiguity, reduced resources
- Financial reality of training and ROI

(Ford, 2019)

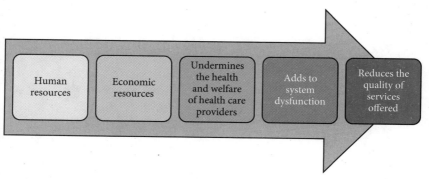

Figure 5-1 The cost of moral injury.

Failing to address moral injury may result in continued loss of valuable health care workers along with the increased chance of harm through clinician error. The long-term impact of failure to address this significant health care concern is The Dystopian future of health care resulting in self-selection into health care of those who will not be harmed by moral injury.

The ethical imperative is to ensure that we are functioning at our optimal level and to recognize when we are not so we can address the issues that are impacting the optimal care we wish to provide and our patients deserve. What is it about clinicians who are not as impacted by the societal pressures that cause Moral Injuty. They are often identified as having "grit" the ability to persevere under difficult circumstances. Those with strong Integrity have internal resilience. GRIT is part of integrity.

Ideas to Consider

1. Ethical risk factors should be considered by:
   a. Therapists who had previous ethical problems.
   b. All therapists in all settings.
   c. Therapists who do not practice with other PTs.
   d. All therapists in private practice.

2. The best way to manage many of the ethical risk factors is:
   a. Critical self-reflection.
   b. Speak to family about them.
   c. Avoid risky patients.
   d. Change work settings.

3. Moral injury is caused by which of the following?
   a. Personal factors.
   b. Patient related factors.
   c. System failures.
   d. Family factors.

CHAPTER 6

Applying Ethical Decision-Making Models in Clinical Practice

The bioethical principles presented in Chapter 1 set the framework for ethical decision-making and will undergird the analysis of the case study that follows demonstrating ethical decision making in the clinical setting. A grasp of these basic principles provides the template for sound clinical decision-making. The actual way in which clinicians arrive at ethical decisions continues to be studied and refined, with a deeper connection to the clinical aspect of decision making. Clearly, ethical and clinical decision-making models must overlap significantly to derive a satisfactory outcome (Dale, 2016; Drumwright, 2015; Kearney and Penque, 2012; Sujdak and Birgitta, 2016).

When physical therapists (PTs) worked under the direction of a medical doctor, many of the opportunities for ethical decision-making were usurped by the hierarchy of that relationship. PTs often recognized an ethical challenge but often felt constrained in their ability to manage it as they did not have the primary responsibility for the situation. The proliferation of direct access states to our current 50 plus the District of Columbia and the change of PT education to the 2017 CAPTE requirement that all programs be at the Doctor of Physical Therapy education level creates a very different professional landscape. PTs must take charge of their ethical decision-making recognizing that the power that provides for independent decision-making also demands collaboration and requires taking responsibility for all the aspects of clinical decisions, this demands that each clinician is accountable for their professional actions. The concept of professional ownership is discussed in more detail in Chapter 3.

THE ETHICAL DECISION-MAKING PROCESS

Ethical decision-making is a challenge to physical therapy professionals, who face both an increase in the number of issues and situations that are increasingly complicated. Ethical decision-making skills are enhanced by studying cases and developing a strategy for facing ethical issues. All practitioners recognize that clinicians don't always have complete control over the situations that confront them. It is the responsibility of the clinician to maintain the focus on the centrality of the patient. When the welfare of the patient is compromised, the healthcare provider is challenged to manage the situation in the patient's best interest (Airth-Kindree and Kirkhorn, 2016; O'Fallon and Butterfield, 2005; Osswald et al., 2009; Rate et al., 2007).

Making decisions is part of everyday living, whether it is deciding what to wear, what to cook for dinner, or what type of vacation to plan. For the most part, these decisions are part of an automatic, and therefore unconscious, process. But there are other decisions, particularly those related to professional practice, that are not automatic. For example, we are often confronted with two equally appropriate choices. Kidder calls this a **right vs. right dilemma**. When evaluating the alternatives, both courses of action have positive and negative elements. Right vs. right is an ethical dilemma, whereas right vs. wrong is identified as a moral temptation. The individual knows the right thing to do, but chooses the action that is wrong (Kidder, 1996). All healthcare providers struggle to establish ethical decision-making standards that provide guidance in a challenging practice environment, and the challenge is not unique to physical therapists. One threat to ethical practice arises from within each profession as a result of materialistic self-interest and from the outside in terms of profit motivation. Another kind of challenge to ethics comes as the result of scientific advances such as mapping of the human genome, which made possible some procedures that raise ethical issues as to whether certain things should be done, such as cloning animals or people, just because they are possible. This type of reasoning always raises the important question of "*Should we take a particular course of action, just because we can?*" This is often the case in end-of-life situations in terms of allowing a person to die whether it be somebody who is elderly, or who has had a catastrophic injury, or in the case of a newborn whose life cannot be sustained without heroic measures.

CLINICAL RELEVANCE

The concept of taking action in a situation just because we can take action is an important overarching concept to consider in ethical decision-making as it speaks to doing what is right for the individual as well as considering the institutional and societal implications of resource utilization. These are decisions that are most often not just the purview of the physical therapist but require an inter-professional approach. This is consistent with the guidance in Principle 3C: Physical therapists shall make judgments within their scope of practice and level of expertise and shall communicate with, collaborate with, or refer to peers or other healthcare professionals when necessary,

A wealth of literature exists on the subject of ethical decision-making. A search of this literature reveals that professionals are inconsistent in ethical decision-making

(Smith et al., 1991; Tymchuk et al., 1982). The literature speaks of the "science" of decision-making but cautions that human limitations result in the inconsistencies that professionals acknowledge in their decision-making skills.

Decision-making is described by Brecke and Garcia (1995) as a course of action that ends uncertainty. The theory they developed requires that the uncertainty associated with the decision must be brought to a level where the decision can be made with confidence. They also place considerable importance on the time that it takes to make a decision. The timeline for decision making can range from a few seconds to several years.

Brecke and Garcia (1995) developed a decision-making process that consisted of four points related to a decision-making timeline. Decisions are made at different points on the timeline, but at any point where action is not taken the decision will ultimately be made by default. Initially, practitioners recognize that there is an opportunity to make a decision. The nature of the decision becomes clearer, and they determine what they will do and then commit to a course of action.

The final point on this continuum is the default point where no intervention on the part of the practitioner will result in a course of action on which they had limited or no input (Brecke and Garcia, 1995). Choosing the default option, or, stated more appropriately, permitting the default option to occur, can be potentially harmful to patients because failure to make a decision carries its own set of ethical concerns. Healthcare providers have a responsibility to protect their patients from harm, and failure to make a decision may place the patient in a potentially harmful situation.

Ethical decision-making is the level that is expected and demanded of professionals. Pellegrino (1993) identifies ethical decision-making as the integration of ethical principles with practical wisdom, enabling healthcare providers to make ethical judgments. Healthcare providers have specific standards and codes that guide practice; these are in the form of codes of ethics and professional practice standards (Newkrug et al., 1996). Codes of ethics are generally broadly written. They help to identify issues, but they are not meant to serve as a methodology for ethical decision-making. To recognize an action and carry out that action requires both knowledge and skill in the art of ethical decision-making.

Patients have the right to expect that their healthcare providers are involving themselves in thoughtful deliberation of ethical issues, with a commitment to take reasonable and rational action. These steps warrant the trust of the patient and society. Unethical, self-serving behaviors result in a loss of trust by patients and their families. According to Dove (1995), the loss of trust could be prevented with training programs that include the application of professional ethics to actual situations.

End-of-life issues, caregiver challenges, and right-to-choose plans of care often become intertwined with ethical issues, and the medical team, patients, and families find that they are confronted by complex ethical decisions. This is made more challenging when the issues involve one or more generations, who may have the same interests at heart but prefer different expressions of those interests.

THE CLASSIC ETHICAL METHODS

Any consideration of ethical analysis would not be complete without looking at the classical framework with ethical analysis. These basic methods are incorporated in some form in most of the ethical decision-making models. These methods answer the "should" questions. What should I do? There are many ethical models, but the most common in healthcare are virtue ethics, consequence-based ethics, and ethics based on principles.

Virtue ethics: Virtues explain "How we should be as healthcare providers." Consider what you think are the ideal characteristics or traits of a physical therapist. Virtues define professional behaviors and often establish the boundaries that provide context for the PT/patient relationship.

Consequence-based ethics: This ethical framework answer the questions "What should I do?" What course of action should I take?

For any course of action, we must determine the "goodness" of that action. This requires looking at the harm benefit ratio. What is the potential for any action to have beneficial consequences vs. the potential harmful consequences? Taking an **"ethical time out"** is often a good plan when considering potential consequences or anticipating potential "collateral damages." An ethical time out is a moment to stop and consider actions, results of inaction, and what you anticipate will be the result, is it the outcome you want?

Principle-based ethics framework: This method also answers the question what should I do? It frames questions using the basic fundamental principles of autonomy, beneficence, Nonmaleficence, and justice. This is also where the APTA Code of Ethics is a most valuable resource.

AN ETHICAL DECISION-MAKING MODEL

There are many models for ethical decision-making that help to organize the thoughts of the individual. Some are quite simplistic. The tilt factor model looks at the choices confronting the individual, with pros and cons defined and with the factors that would change the decision indicated as tilt factors. This simple model does not truly guide the practitioners' actions, but it does help to frame the question.

Among the many models available is one offered by Kornblau and Starling (2000). This template provides the practitioner with guidance for collecting information about the problem, the facts of the situation, the identification of interested parties, and the nature of their interest: Is it professional, personal, business, economic, intellectual, or societal? The practitioner is then encouraged to determine if an ethical question is involved and if there is a violation of the code of ethics of their profession, or if there is a potential affront to their moral, social, or religious values. This model also demands that any potential legal issue such as malpractice, or a practice-act infringement, be identified. The practitioner is encouraged to gather more information if it is needed to make an appropriate decision. This is the point where the healthcare provider is encouraged to brainstorm potential actions and then analyze the course of the chosen action.

Another method of ethical decision-making that is increasingly popular with physical therapists is the Realm, Individual Process, Situation (RIPS) model (Swisher et al., 2005). The steps in ethical decision-making, which use the RIPS model, bring forward many of the aspects of a problem confronting the interdisciplinary team.

This method essentially involves five steps. To better illustrate the ethical decision-making process, we will work through a case that involves issues of utilization. You will see that the three primary components of the RIPS model are implemented in the case discussion below.

Case Example 1

TOO MUCH OF A GOOD THING

Adapted, with permission, from Kirsch N. Ethical decision making: Application of a problem-solving model. *Top Geriatr Rehabil.* 2009;25(4):282–291.

Mr. Markham is 82 years old, and he has been in relatively good health. He does have high blood pressure, and eight years ago he had bypass surgery. He lives with his 79-year-old wife in the two-story home they have owned for more than 40 years. He is retired from an executive position at a large manufacturing company. His primary insurance is Medicare.

Two weeks ago, he awakened disoriented in the middle of the night and fell as he tried to get out of bed to use the bathroom. His wife called 911 and he was taken to the hospital, where it was determined he had sustained a right CVA with a resulting left hemiplegia. His course in the hospital was complicated by an unexplained fever. When he had been fever-free for 48 hours it was determined that he could be discharged to a subacute facility to begin rehabilitation.

Mr. Markham looks forward to starting rehabilitation but is very tired and finds it difficult to tolerate the 30 minutes of therapy he is receiving in the hospital. He has only been out of bed for 20 minutes at a time and was exhausted afterward. He and his family are assured by staff that he will continue to get stronger each day.

At the subacute facility, he is evaluated by physical therapy (PT), occupational therapy (OT), and speech therapy. He is found to have no speech deficits and no cognitive deficits other than mild confusion, which is steadily clearing. His entire program will thus consist of physical therapy and occupational therapy. Following evaluation, he is placed on Tim's caseload for PT and Casey's caseload for OT.

Mr. Markham is assigned a very high level RUG rehab (Resource Utilization Group, under Medicare Part A) and Tim and Casey plan his program around the required 500 minutes of therapy in seven days required for this RUG level. He is to receive over an hour of service per day, seven days a week.

The first day Tim sees Mr. Markham, the patient is begging to return to his room after 15 minutes. His blood pressure has dropped and he had tachycardia. He is diaphoretic and becoming increasingly lethargic. Tim returns Mr. Markham to his room, recognizing that he will have to make up the time in the afternoon. Casey sees Mr. Markham after lunch and, though he wants to cooperate, Mr. Markham cannot do more than 20 minutes before he is having difficulty keeping his head up.

When Tim arrives to take Mr. Markham to PT in the afternoon, he finds him asleep and difficult to rouse. Tim and Casey confer at the end of the day and find that between them they saw Mr. Markham for 35 minutes. They report the situation to the rehab supervisor, who reminds them of the importance of achieving the full 500 minutes and tells them to be sure to include the missed time over the rest of the week. He reminds them that if Mr. Markham cannot participate in therapy, he may have to be discharged from the subacute facility to a nursing home.

Tim and Casey wonder if Mr. Markham should be at the assigned RUG level, the second highest level of therapy. They are concerned that, if they push him to achieve the level in which he has been placed, they could compromise his fragile medical condition. On the other hand, if he cannot do the program they have designed for him and he is sent to a nursing home, there is little chance of his doing well enough to ever return home. Tim and Casey are very uncomfortable with the situation in which they find themselves.

The following day they rearrange their schedules, switching a few patients to afford Mr. Markham more advantageous times of the day. He does a bit better but still cannot achieve even 45 minutes of combined time. Tim and Casey approach their supervisor again and ask for a decrease in the RUG level for Mr. Markham. Once again they are told to make it work. The lower rehab category does not have sufficient time to justify a subacute stay for this patient.

From experience Tim and Casey recognize that "make it work" means they need to provide the minutes of treatment, but they cannot rationalize placing this patient at risk to meet the minutes. They believe their supervisors do not share their concern and feel that their professional values could easily be compromised as they balance their desire to act with nonmaleficence (not harming the patient) while maintaining veracity (being truthful regarding the treatment rendered).

APPLYING A MODIFIED RIPS MODEL TO THE CASE

Through "Tim" and "Casey" we will work through this situation using a multi-faceted ethical decision-making model that combines the work of Kornblau and Starling (2000) and Kidder (1996), and the RIPS model developed by Swisher and colleagues (2005). The following model sequence, helps to establish a logical format for integrating the RIPS model with the work of Kornblau, Starling, and Kidder. It also builds a framework for self-reflection and professional growth.

A Model Sequence for Ethical Decision Making and Professional Development

Step 1: Recognize and define the ethical issues: Apply The RIPs Model:
Realm
Individual process
Situation

Step 2: Reflect
1. facts and contextual information?
2. major stakeholders?
3. Consider the legal requirements and ethical concerns
4. What do the core documents of the profession have to say
5. Are any of the five tests for right vs. wrong situation-positive?
   (legal test, stench test, front-page test, Mom test, professional ethics test)

Step 3: Decide the right thing to do:
Consider Rules based, ends based and care based contexts.
Consider the ethical frameworks to resolve the issue:
1) Virtue Based ethics: How should I be?
2) Consequence Based ethics: What are the intended and unintended consequences and who is impacted?
3) Principle Based ethics: Which ethical principle(s) apply to my situation:
   a. Autonomy
   b. Beneficence
   c. Non-maleficence
   d. Justice
   e. Veracity

Step 4: Implement, Evaluate and Reassess the course of action.
What steps should you take?
What resources do you need to implement your plan?
Consider the results of your actions.

Step 5: Personal growth and reflection
- What did you as a professional learn from this situation? How can you apply what you have learned to subsequent situations?
- What are your strengths and weaknesses in terms of the individual processes of Moral sensitivity, judgment, motivation and courage.
- Is there a need for you to plan professional activities to grow in any of the individual processes or the ability to apply the three ethical frameworks?

Step 1: Recognize and Define the Ethical Issue

Realm

As presented in the model we will first recognize and define the type of ethical issue we are confronted with. Into which of the three realms presented in the model does this case fall?—individual, organizational/institutional, or societal.

This situation falls into the institutional realm. The care of the patient is being dictated by institutional policy. There is also a societal component here because the policies dictated by a third-party payer (Medicare), care is determined largely on payment parameters, but a professional must weigh treatment outcomes vs. treatment options. In this case, it appears that payment is driving practice, not practice driving payment.

Individual Process

What does the situation require of Tim and Casey? What individual process is most appropriate? According to the model there are four components to the individual process. To manage an ethical issue, all four components of the process must come into play at some point, although there is no particular order in which the components are handled. The four components are defined as follows.

Moral sensitivity: This involves recognizing that there is an issue and being aware of its impact. Tim and Casey recognize that this is an ethical issue. They cannot rationalize treating Mr. Markham at a level that he cannot tolerate; not only will it lack benefit, but it also has a high probability of being detrimental to him.

Moral judgment: The individual considers possible actions and what the effect will be on all parties. Tim and Casey recognize that, while they are right to insist that their patient not be forced into therapy he cannot tolerate, if Mr. Markham cannot participate fully in the program at the level it has been set, he risks being discharged to a lower level of care or to home without the benefit of the rehab program he needs. Tim and Casey are torn because they believe that Mr. Markham just needs some time to build up his endurance, but they cannot document treatment not rendered. Will their honesty result in his loss of services?

Moral motivation: This is the force that compels the individual to consider possible courses of action. Casey and Tim are not willing to compromise their integrity or their loyalty to their patient. They want him to get the services to which he is entitled, but they also want to protect him. Their supervisors appear to see only the financial ramifications of Mr. Markham's lack of treatment. Tim and Casey are faced with falsifying minutes to protect his treatment program, treating him at a level that he cannot tolerate, or risking early discharge by treating him to his tolerance and documenting appropriately. While they support each other in their ethical decision making, they do not feel they are getting much support from their superiors.

Moral courage: This is a measure of ego strength, the strength to take action to correct a wrong. It is interchangeable with moral character. Tim and Casey feel strongly that Mr. Markham should be given a lower RUG level, realistically, a rehab high-level—until he can tolerate more therapy. Administration does not support this view, but Tim and Casey are very emphatic. They cite the literature supporting this more moderate approach and attempt to get their supervisor to understand their discomfort with the treatment protocol. The treatment plan put in place by administration compromises the autonomy to which they are obligated by the practice acts for each of their disciplines.

Moral failure: This is deficiency in any of the four components, the failure to recognize that an issue exists, the inability to plan a course of action, the lack of motivation to take action, and the inability to follow through on the action. The supervisors and administration in the facility are subject to moral failure with deficiencies in multiple areas.

Moral potency: This is the element that, when absent, results in action not being taken. As a relative newcomer, moral potency is a concept we have to grow into (Schaubroeck et al., 2010).

Situation

The model presents five possible types of ethical situations for us to identify. What type of an ethical situation is this: a problem, a distress, a dilemma, a temptation, or a silence?

An ethical problem: The practitioner is confronted with challenges or threats to their own moral duties and values. This results in a need to reflect on a course of action.

An ethical distress: The focus is on the practitioner. The practitioner knows what action should be taken, but there is a barrier in the way of doing what is right. The individuals experience some discomfort because they are prevented from being the kinds of persons they want to be or doing what they know is right.

An ethical dilemma: This type of problem involves two or more morally correct courses of action where only one can be followed. In choosing one course of action over another, the practitioner is doing something right and wrong at the same time.

An ethical temptation: This involves two or more courses of action, one that is morally correct and one that is morally incorrect but, for reasons determined by the practitioner, they consciously choose the incorrect course of action.

Silence: The practitioner chooses to ignore the problem, and takes no action. So, from the above we see that Tim and Casey are faced with an ethical distress.

They know the correct action they wish to take but they are unable to take that action because of institutional constraints.

Ideas to Consider

1. Right vs. wrong may be a moral temptation, but right vs. right is:
   a. The best of both worlds.
   b. An ethical dilemma.
   c. A chance for correct action.
   d. A political brawl.

2. When PTs act to correct a situation, they are exhibiting:
   a. Moral sensitivity.
   b. Moral judgment.
   c. Moral motivation.
   d. Moral courage.

3. When PTs decide on a line of action, they are exhibiting:
   a. Moral sensitivity.
   b. Moral judgment.
   c. Moral motivation.
   d. Moral courage.

4. When PTs recognize an ethical problem but take no action, it is called:
   a. An ethical distress.
   b. An ethical dilemma.
   c. An ethical temptation.
   d. An ethical silence.

Step 2: Reflect

In the model the additional steps two, three and four, give us the opportunity to gather more information necessary to make a decision.

What else do we need to know about the situation, the patient, and the family? Who are the Interested parties (stakeholders) in addition to Mr. Markham, the patient, and the health-care practitioners, Tim and Casey. The following people are also stakeholders, or potential stakeholders:

- The patient's wife
- The institution, and the supervisor
- Other healthcare providers
- The insurance company
- The licensing board charged with protecting the public
- The professional association and its code of ethics

What Are the Consequences of Action?

Determining a plan of care is based on the assessment of the patient and available resources for treatment. In this situation, the assessment indicates the need for care and the resources are available to the patient, but the rehab professionals have their plan of care dictated by the institution/third-party reimbursement. The professionals find the care to be unreasonable and potentially harmful; however, if they refuse to carry out the care as it is proposed, they may endanger the patient's access to care in their facility.

What Are the Consequences of Inaction?

The members of the rehab team understand that failure to question the plan of care and, instead, attempting to impose the RUG parameters on this patient may place the patient in danger. Mr. Markham is not medically stable enough to manage care at the level they are being forced to deliver it. In many cases, this is a time-sensitive issue because the patient may be able in the future to benefit from the care, but the current level of recovery is insufficient to tolerate it. Rehabilitation professionals often find themselves caught between what they have determined is appropriate for the patient and external pressures regarding the delivery of care.

The last step of the reflection phase is associated with a proposal by Rushworth Kidder in *How Good People Make Tough Choices* (Kidder, 1996). Kidder initially proposed a four-standard test. Later, a fifth standard was added because the Kidder test was being applied to professional ethics. A code of ethics/professional guidance check was incorporated into the test.

Kidder Test Adapted to Markham Case

1. The Legal Test

- Are any laws potentially broken?
- What does the state practice act say about providing inappropriate care?
- What does the practice act demand of licensed professionals as to their autonomy and their individual responsibility to make decisions that are not dictated or controlled by other sources?
- Does the potential exist that the rehab professionals are culpable if they cannot make the minutes required, and the care is being billed at the RUG level?
- How close do they come to billing in a potentially fraudulent manner?

2. The Stench Test

Does the situation feel right, or does it stink? The uncomfortable feeling of a professional when integrity is challenged produces a positive response to the stench test. The individual knows that "it stinks." In good conscious, professionals cannot pretend the situation does not exist or is beyond their control.

3. The Front Page Test

Is the potential publicity something you would not like to have on the front page? Healthcare providers generally take pride in the work they do. Positive publicity is welcomed by most professionals, but negative publicity reflects badly on all practitioners and is poorly received by the healthcare community. Negative publicity does considerable harm because it diminishes public trust. Imagine the headline in our case: "Patient welfare compromised in a revenue enhancement scheme."

4. The Mom Test

The final Kidder test looks at the background of the individual, recognizing that much of our ethical decision making has strong foundations in our upbringing, reflecting the value system of those who influenced us along the way. Kidder calls this the "mom" test, but it is broader than the values instilled by your mother. It incorporates not just parental guidance but also those mentors, teachers, and colleagues who have influenced your values as a professional. The mom test integrates personal integrity with the professional values that every healthcare professional brings to the situation.

If the action you are contemplating would not be acceptable to those who helped you develop your value system, you must consider other actions more consistent with the values that you hold to be important. If this requires a change in behavior, then you are faced with an ethical challenge to develop a course of action that is different and would be acceptable. In this case, continuing to treat this patient despite Tim's and Casey's concerns about Mr. Markham's well-being would not pass the mom test.

5. The Professional Values Test

This is the element that was added to the Kidder test, which was originally devised for society in general and not for professionals. What guidance do we get from professional standards? The physical therapist involved with the care of this patient has access to guidance from the APTA Code of Ethics (2017a). Codes and other professional documents help individuals determine what their responsibility is to the patient. The APTA Code of Ethics and Standards of Ethical Conduct for the Physical Therapist Assistant were completely revised effective July 1, 2010.

Consider the following guidance from the Code of Ethics:

- **3A:** Physical therapists shall demonstrate independent and objective professional judgment in the patient/client's best interest in all practice settings.
- **7A:** Physical therapists shall promote practice environments that support autonomous and accountable professional judgments.

The case made by the therapists on behalf of the patient contained current evidence and was substantiated by the literature. This is consistent with Principle **3B:** Physical therapists shall demonstrate professional judgment informed by professional standards. Evidenced by (including current literature and established best practice) practitioner experience and patient/client values (APTA, 2017b).

If the situation does not pass the Kidder test, there is no need to go any further. The only question remaining is whether the healthcare professional has the moral courage to follow through and take appropriate action. Action in this case must be taken in order to preserve professional integrity (Kirsch, 2006). For Tim and Casey, taking action to place their patient's needs above those of the institution would be more consistent with their professional values.

Step 3: Decide the Right Thing to Do

Step 3 presumes that all the factual material has been investigated and the individual is now ready to make a decision. The adapted Kidder assesses the factual information against the five standards of law, stench, front page, parent/mentor, and professional guidance.

If any of the Kidder tests is positive, action must be taken. Even if the situation passes the Kidder test, there may still be an ethical issue to consider. At that point, the information you have gathered must be considered in view of three classical approaches to ethical decision making: rule-based, ends-based, or care-based.

Rule-Based Approach

People who take the rule-based approach follow that which they think everybody else should follow. These are the rules, duties, and obligations already in place (Gabard and Martin, 2003). The procedures, techniques, and methods are what would be considered the "standard of care." It is not hard to conceive of an approach that would apply selected parameters to care rendered and clearly define certain limits. In addition, objective measurements are available to provide guidance about the ethical dilemma of over-treating a medically fragile patient in order to qualify for care from which he cannot yet benefit. Standardized assessments—such as those for blood pressure, heart rate, oxygen absorption, reaction to exercise—provide objective measurements that are easily applied and interpreted.

Applying a rules-based approach to our patient's situation would ensure that care not be rendered to the patient if he could not tolerate it. Note that this approach does not protect the patient against the situation where care is no longer available because he cannot meet the standard.

Ends-Based Approach

Those using the ends-based approach do whatever produces the greatest good for the most people. The analysis of the action and the resulting outcomes looks at the good and harm for all of the stakeholders, not just the patient (Sugarman, 2000). An ends-based approach looks more at the general good for society and less at the individual's needs. This would be the least likely application in our case.

Care-Based Approach

Those using the care-based approach follow the Golden Rule ("Do unto others as you would have them do unto you") (Gabard and Martin, 2003). Situations are resolved according to relationships and concern for others. It is difficult for healthcare providers to remove themselves from the situation completely, but they can recall a personal experience or another patient-care situation that reminds them how important it is to integrate the ethic of care into the entire patient-care situation. Step 3 encourages the rehabilitation professional to implement the decision made. There is reasonable evidence that this will resolve the issue. But implementing a plan does not conclude the ethical decision-making process. Each situation provides an opportunity to learn more and to develop a workable plan for managing future situations.

Choose one or more of the ethical frameworks:

Value based: How should I be

Consequence Based and Principle based both asking how should I act.

Step 4: Implement, Evaluate, and Reassess

It is the responsibility of the professional to reflect on the chosen course of action and consider any steps needed to avoid this type of ethical situation in the future. The responsibility to modify behavior lies not only with the individual but also with the institution. The situation confronting Tim and Casey points to the difficulty of implementing plans of care that are not at the discretion of the treating practitioner. The patient's entire team needs to make the treatment a collaborative effort. To effect the most positive outcome, this includes the patient and family. For the team to work as a cohesive unit, there must be mutual understanding and respect for the unique contribution of each team member and the way in which that contribution can benefit the approach to the patient (Badawi, 2016; Keehan et al., 2008; McCarthy and Gastmans, 2015).

Step 5: Personal Growth and Reflection

It is the responsibility of every professional to determine what they learned from the situation and how they can apply it going forward. For the Markham case the professional might answer the following questions.

- What was learned from the case involving Mr. Markham and his plan of care? For Tim and Casey, they confirmed their professional responsibility to be autonomous practitioners. They also recognized the constraints they have working in a setting that does not necessarily respect that responsibility.
- What are the strengths and weaknesses of the practitioner with regard to the individual processes? Does the individual exhibit moral sensitivity, judgment, motivation, and courage? Tim and Casey exhibited moral sensitivity, judgment, and motivation. We don't know the outcome of this scenario. We do know that moral courage would require overt action on their part to protect their patient.
- Is the profession mature enough to have developed the ability to move ahead in recognizing the necessity for moral potency? (Schaubroeck et al., 2010; Tenbrunsel and Messick, 2008; Tenbrunsel and Smith-Crowe, 2008).
- If the provider needs to develop one or all of these skills, what type of professional activities would help to accomplish this? Ethical reasoning can be taught (Handelsman, 1986). The best method for teaching ethical decision-making skills is through case studies (Reuben et al., 2004). Teaching ethics does diminish the uncertainty that is inherent in ethical decision-making. Seeking the opportunity to further develop these skills is critical to sound ethical decision making.

- Was the outcome what was expected? Was there any collateral damage? When confronted with an ethical situation, we may carry some preconceived concepts about what may result. It is important to look back at the outcome and compare it to what we anticipated. This is particularly important when collateral damage may be worse than the initial situation. Preventing collateral damage is always preferable to trying to ameliorate them after the fact. A thorough review of collateral damages—similar to a risk/benefit ratio—may be enough to suggest mechanisms to prevent them in the future. Elger and Harding (2002) suggest that if collateral damage cannot be prevented there has to be an assessment to determine if the damage is worse than what would occur as a result of the ethical breech.

The previous case was analyzed extensively. We will look at the following case with a more clinically friendly approach.

Case Example 2

STEPPING OVER THE LINE?

Adapted, with permission, from Kirsch N. *Ethics in Practice PT: The Magazine of Physical Therapy*. Ahead of print February 2017.

Jim makes a point to sign up for at least one student physical therapist a year. While it takes a lot of time, he feels strongly that it is a professional responsibility. He gratefully remembers his clinical instructors while he was in school and wants to "pay it forward" providing a quality experience for a student. The other therapists in the large rehabilitation hospital where he works also consider the student program a significant way to be engaged with the profession. Tom, his new third-year student from State, is starting his final clinical rotation. Jim and Tom hit it off immediately and Jim begins to orient Tom to the patient's and the routine at the hospital, generally a rather steep learning curve in this very busy clinical environment where every patient is complex. It is not unusual for students assigned to this facility to have difficulty. It is known to be quite challenging. While the days are busy, the two men find a few minutes to discuss the sports headlines and banter about the prospects for the upcoming season. Unfortunately, Jim finds that Tom is not prepared for the neurological case load that Jim is treating. Jim is willing to help Tom and both men come in early and stay late but Tom is still struggling. He is in contact with the school, and the Director of Clinical Education visited the facility to work with Tom and Jim. They determine that a learning contract should be put in place, so it is very clear to all what is expected of Tom to successfully complete this clinical rotation. Though he was having difficulty and Jim still was unable to give him the caseload he should be carrying, they still had a very good working relationship. During lunch break on Friday, Jim shares with Tom that he and his wife are moving from their apartment to their new house and one of his friends that was going to help with the move was sick. Jim suddenly looks at Tom and without seemingly stopping to think he says to Tom, "hey I've taught you everything you need to know about body mechanics, can you give me a hand?" Tom did have weekend plans, but he is pretty sure that everybody will understand the importance of helping out his CI, he sees it as an opportunity to help his CI who has been so good to him ... yet as he gives it more thought he is concerned that it could appear that he just trying to "butter up" his CI. He doesn't think that it is right, but he didn't see he had much choice ... so Tom willingly agrees to help out, spending both Saturday and Sunday as Jim's "right-hand man." Monday morning Tom and two of the other students who were at the clinical site compared their weekend activities. When Tom shares with them that he helped Jim all weekend, they exchange a knowing glance, passing the comment "that should insure a passing grade" before going off to start their day.

While on the surface this may appear not too much of an ethical breech, there are some rather significant boundary crossings that occur and are easily extrapolated to other situations when you consider the many potential ramifications.

Recognize and Define the Ethical Issues

In which **realm** does this occur? This is occurring in the individual realm. It is a situation occurring between the two men Jim the CI and Tom his eager but struggling student.

The **individual process** for Jim is moral sensitivity; he fails to recognize that he is placing the student in a difficult situation. For Tom, he is faced with a moral judgment: how will his willingness to help appear ... and if he declines how will that appear?

Ethical situation. This is a moral problem for Jim, but it is a potential distress for Tom as he attempts to determine if the decision that he is making is appropriate. It could also be considered a moral temptation as Tom, the student, does recognize that he is stepping into a situation that is beyond the therapist–student relationship, but he does stand potentially to benefit from it, and he needs all the help he can get.

Reflect and Take Action

Not every step of the reflection must be completed in a shorter ethical analysis; the practitioner chooses those aspects of the analysis that will provide the information they need.

1. Who are the stakeholders? Defining the stakeholders helps the therapist reflect on the broader nature of this case—it is not just Jim and Tom involved, it

certainly impacts patients currently, and in the future if Tom is not competent to treat, this will impact both the individual patient's and the credibility of the profession. It also impacts the school. As they are aware of the difficulty he is having, can they continue to rely on the objectivity of the CI Jim? The school relies on the objectivity of the clinical instructors in determining if students are prepared for clinical practice.

2. What are the possible consequences (intended and unintended)? The possible consequence could be that the dual relationship that Jim created could result in his evaluating Tom using a different standard than he would use for other students that he is not as close with.

3. What are the relevant laws, duties, and obligations? He has an obligation to be fair, and he did exert some undue pressure on Tom, which is explained in the Code of Ethics: Principle 4B:

4. *Ethical principles.* The following principle of the Code of Ethics for the Physical Therapist offers Jim guidance in his decision-making process:

- Principle **4B**: Physical therapists shall not exploit persons over whom they have supervisory, evaluative or other authority.

Ideas to Consider

5. When action is taken based on the standard of care, it is:
   a. Care based.
   b. Rule based.
   c. Ends based.
   d. Ethics based.

6. When action is taken based on achieving the greatest good, it is:
   a. Care based.
   b. Rule based.
   c. Ends based.
   d. Ethics based.

7. The final step of a professional in ethical decision-making is:
   a. Implement, evaluate, and reassess.
   b. Recognize and reflect.
   c. Decide and implement.
   d. File a report.

CHAPTER 7

Practicing Ethically in a Digital World

In the first edition of this book telehealth was addressed in the "future" chapter. While many of the important components of telehealth were in place at the time very little telehealth was being done and it was anticipated that at least another decade would pass before telehealth became a potential mainstream way in which to deliver physical therapy services. A global pandemic changed the practice landscape bringing telehealth into mainstream practice with the accompanying ethical considerations.

Telehealth is defined as care at a distance: Telehealth is about access; Access to providers and providers' access to patients. In a "hands-on" profession such as physical therapy, there is understandable concern about this care delivery model (American Telehealth Association, 2023). The basic ethical principles prevail regardless of setting, and telehealth is just that, another physical therapy practice setting. A remote expert is a wonderful adjunct but does not completely replace the provider who is on site. Practice must still maintain the centrality of the patient as a whole when determining the optimal location for the delivery of health care through telehealth (Cheshire, 2017).

Physical therapy can be delivered through telehealth in several different formats.

Pure Telerehabilitation consists of services provided completely remotely. There is also a hybrid model in which the initial evaluation is done in person and subsequent sessions remotely. Another model of care delivery is either synchronous where communication is occurring in real time or asynchronous where sensors are utilized to deliver data which is responded to by the therapist at a later time. The least effective type of telerehab is telecommunication only, voice and no video, while there may be times this is adequate most of the time it is not an effective methodology for the delivery of physical therapy services.

When considering telehealth as a viable setting there are seven things to consider.

1. Clinician competence.
2. Right person, right place, right time.
3. Patient safety.
4. Legality.
5. Privacy.
6. Confidentiality.
7. Evidence-based support.

Clinician competence: Though not restricted to clinicians with experience only individual clinicians must carefully assess their skill set and comfort level with delivering care remotely and managing the treatment venue including the effective use of technology. (Principle 3C, 6A)

Right person, right place, right time: Telehealth is not a replacement for the delivery of optimal care, it should never be considered "better than nothing." Not all patients are right for telehealth delivery, or they are not in the place for the care they need or not in the right time considering their recovery. (Principle 3A)

Patient safety: is critically important, Is the home environment safe for the patient and care givers. Can the therapist adequately assess that patient or develop interventions that are appropriate and ensure the patient's safety as they participate. Consider not just the obvious risks but the hidden risks as well. (Principle 3A)

Legality: Telehealth permits access, but it also blurs the jurisdictional boundaries and therapists must be cognizant of where the patient is physically located at the time to make sure that they can legally practice in that state. In addition, the PT must know whether Telehealth practice by physical therapists and physical therapist assistants is legal in that jurisdiction. The PT compact has been developing simultaneously with the growth of telehealth and has been quite beneficial in making access more readily available. (Principle 5A)

Privacy: In every setting, patient privacy is of paramount importance. Each setting has its own unique challenge, but telehealth has an entirely new set of challenges in terms of the platform used and making sure that it is HIPAA compliant. Privacy is more difficult to guarantee when the patient is at home as others may be in the area without the knowledge of the PT. (Principle 2E)

Confidentiality: Similar to the challenges of privacy, maintaining confidentiality by only using HIPAA compliant platforms protects the patient and the clinician. Confidentiality is one of the oldest ethical duties and attributed to Hippocrates, it is well established in the principle of autonomy. (Principle 2E)

Evidence-based support for treatment: Telehealth in the U.S. is in its early stages and there is little information to use to compare the outcomes between Telehealth and traditional face to face treatment. The demands for efficacy of treatment rationale are unchanged regardless of venue. We must begin to collect, study and disseminate information to better inform practice. (Principles 3B, 6C)

In reality none of these considerations are exclusive to telehealth care, they are things that should be considered all the time when determining what patients need and how to best deliver care.

It is important to remember that the relationship between the patient and the clinician is unchanged by the method of care delivery. A patient–clinician relationship must be established, and it is built on a foundation of trust. Making that personal connection is more difficult in a telehealth encounter but care must be taken to establish it early, as effective communication will depend on this early connection. As in any relationship the clinician must also be aware of any potential conflict of interest in the choice of treatment venue. Will the patient derive an equivalent value from a telehealth visit vs. an inpatient visit? Clinician experience is very beneficial for a telehealth visit, though there are no restrictions at this time based on experience. When treating in person there may be certain tasks you can delegate to an aide. When treating remotely your aide is technology. You must self-assess as to whether you are competent using technology and able to help trouble shoot with your patient to achieve optimal results. The ethical responsibility to know yourself, your personal strengths and weaknesses so as to cause no harm is critical (Nebeker et al, 2018, Nebeker et al 2019, Nebeker, 2020).

Examining the delivery of a PT encounter via telehealth is done through both a clinical and an ethical lens. When we think about the virtues that we associate with our Code of Ethics each one of them should be considered when considering a telehealth encounter (Figure 7-1).

The optimal treatment environment speaks to compassion and professional duty. Choosing the environment that is best is not just most convenient calls upon integrity and altruism. All health care requires collaboration and accountability and making services as accessible as possible is our social responsibility. The over-arching virtue of Excellence is constantly at the forefront of our decision making in determining the type of care and the location of that care.

Before we embark on a care path, applying a consequentialism framework is an excellent way to evaluate the rightness or wrongness of the action and to anticipate what could potentially go wrong and what as a clinician I may have not considered.

Finally applying a principle-based approach:

Autonomy: Have the patient and caregivers been given sufficient information to make an informed decision about the options for telehealth vs. in person?

Beneficience: Is the treatment in the best interest of the patient?

Non-maleficence: Will treating via telehealth potentially cause harm?

Justice: Can we make these services available to all of our patients for whom they may be necessary?

Veracity: Are we truthful and honest about what patients should expect from a telehealth visit?

There are some heightened responsibilities that the clinician has when engaging in a telehealth visit that are necessary to ensure the safety of the patient. It is essential that you establish at each visit the address where the patient is at for that particular encounter. In case of an emergency, you have to know where the patient is to get help in a timely manner. This cannot be done just once as the patient can easily be in a different location. You also need to establish that they are in a safe place to participate. Know who is with the patient and make sure the patient is comfortable with them being there, you also want to know who is with the patient who may be able to assist with their program and also in case of emergency. If the patient is a minor and particularly if they are younger or if they are a vulnerable adult a telehealth visit though convenient, may not be the most beneficial for the patient.

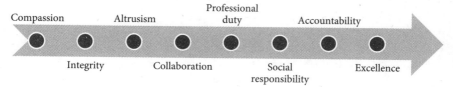

Figure 7-1 Physical Therapy Core Values

Case Study

Jill has been treating Mary for two weeks. Ten weeks ago, Mary underwent a left total hip replacement using a posterior approach. Mary was had strict precautions not to bend her trunk beyond 90 degrees and cross her legs. Jill has been very careful to help Mary abide by her restrictions during her telehealth sessions. Jill was at the airport waiting for her flight, when her office manager texted to remind her of Mary's telehealth appointment in five minutes, an appointment that Jill forgot. Only having a smart phone, Jill decided to do the session using her smart phone. She did not tell Mary she was at the airport using a smart phone. During Mary's exercises, Jill was distracted by the people and noise at the airport and was unable to closely monitor Mary. Suddenly, she heard Mary scream and fall in pain, the cause of which later revealed was a posterior hip dislocation.

Recognize and Define the Ethical Issues

In which **realm** does this occur? It is occurring in the individual realm between the patient and the therapist. The **individual process** for Jill was a moral failure. She failed to recognize the potential consequences of her providing care in a less than optimal set of circumstances. The **situation** was an ethical temptation. Jill should have considered whether or not she could provide optimal care for the patient under the circumstances, the safest course of action would have been to reschedule.

Reflect

Jill was not fully transparent with the patient. She did not let her know where she was, or what she was using for the call. She did not consider the potential consequences of her action and the risk that put the patient at because of her location. She certainly could not ensure that patient privacy could be maintained or patient confidentiality. She was not using a HIPAA compliant platform.

Code of Ethics Guidance

Principle 2A: Physical therapists shall adhere to the core values of the profession and shall act in the best interest of patients/clients over the interest of the physical therapist.

Principle 3D: Physical therapists shall not engage in conflicts of interest that interfere with professional judgment.

Principle 5A: Physical therapists shall comply with applicable local, state, and federal laws and regulations.

Digital Health

Digital health is a relative newcomer to the health care industry, but it has progressed so rapidly in the past few years that it needs to be addressed not for its potential future impact but rather for the impact it has now and the many ethical issues that it raises (Cheshire, 2017). Digital health combines several different technology-based health care delivery methods. Telecommunications and mobile communication technology coupled with wearable technology provide what are called rehabilitation and health promotion services. These services are being delivered in different formats. Some are traditional synchronous telerehabilitation with licensed therapists interacting with the patient and the data they are producing. Others focus on asynchronous data-driven programs that do not establish a traditional patient clinician relationship utilizing bots and artificial intelligence or untrained health coaches to create algorithms based on movement data supplied by the patient utilizing primarily wearable technology. Physical Therapists and Physical Therapist Assistants providing these services must be very cognizant of what they are providing and to whom and what the expectations are of their services and the use of their license number. The attraction of these services to large insurance companies is of course cost savings without any data to show that the services provided are as effective as those that are delivered in person or in synchronous telehealth session. Clinicians need to be cognizant of their ethical responsibility to note individuals who do not have conditions appropriate for digital treatment. The physical therapist and the PTA also need to practice within their scope and within the law, meeting the evaluation, documentation, and plan of care requirements within their jurisdiction. Awareness of breaches of term and title protection are extremely important not just on the individual level for the patient but also on the societal level when patients believe that the service that they were provided was physical therapy when it was not. Patients with poor outcomes who believe they received physical therapy are unfortunately not going to pursue professional physical therapy services. The algorithms developed using artificial intelligence (AI) are questionable and the information may be premature in its usefulness. The data is insufficient to derive a plan of care without human/machine interaction. To develop programs based solely on AI would not rise to the standard of care expected of a physical therapist. Potential harm increases significantly because of the likelihood that the data is not robust enough to make appropriate clinical judgments. The use of AI and digital technology has tremendous potential for greater access to care and improved clinical outcomes, but artificial intelligence is not quite ready to provide valuable information to inform the plan of care for a patient. Ultimately AI will be a part of the decision-making process as appropriate freeing up the physical therapist to do the aspects of care that demand human interaction. The introduction of new technology requires that the physical therapist do an ethical analysis using the three frameworks, First from a principles perspective, at question is whether the the patient's autonomy is respected and do they have enough information to give informed consent using digital health. Will the proposed intervention help the patient (beneficience) or is there a chance it could cause harm (non-maleficence). An assessment of the virtues of excellence, social responsibility and accountability can help guide the physical therapist in determining what technology they would like to institute. Finally, a consequence-based analysis should define the harm benefit ratio of becoming involved in digital health. The nature of healthcare, the treatment of vulnerable populations makes it even more important to be very mindful and careful in introducing new technology. The technology should stand a multifaceted test to determine if it truly is of benefit to the patient. In addition to the ethics test there are other models to make a sound determination regarding the use of a newer methodology. Pagoto and Nebeker (2019) introduced a digital health decision-making framework that works well with our ethical decision-making frameworks. The framework consists of five domains, (1) Participant privacy, (2) Risks and benefits, (3) Access and usability, (4) Data management and (5) Ethical principles. The five domains are designed to have a relationship between them that intersects to help determine what is in the best interest of patients.

Case Study

George is a new graduate. He is working in a PT owned private practice where he did one of his clinical placements and receiving great mentorship. He recently attended a professional meeting and was excited to be networking with colleagues from all over the country. While at the conference he was approached by one of the large digital health companies. They invited him out to dinner to discuss some of the opportunities available to him in the rapidly evolving digital marketplace. George was intrigued by the possibilities that lay ahead with digital health and curious to learn more about how it may be utilized in the future. Mike the CEO of the digital start-up was not a PT but was very knowledgeable about the field and very enthusiastic about how digital health specifically for musculoskeletal issues could revolutionize the delivery of PT services, improving access and therefore outcomes. George was particularly intrigued by the opportunity to pick up some digital health patients as a "side gig" that he could do on his own time, it would not interfere with his regular schedule, but it would certainly provide some much-needed cash to start paying down that hefty loan that got him through PT school. Mike assured George he could do as many or as few patients as he would like to have. He will review the patient questionnaire and choose the appropriate exercises to load on the tablet that the patient receives. As long as the patient was following through with their program, he would not have to have additional contact with them though he will still be on payroll as a consultant, but the contact will primarily be through the health coach. George was certainly intrigued but could not help feeling that he needed to do a bit more investigation as something was making him feel a bit uncomfortable.

Recognize and Define the Ethical Issues

While initially he thought the **realm** would be individual as he considered the impact of digital physical therapy, he recognized that the appropriate realm is societal. For many people this may be their only contact with physical therapy. Is what they are receiving truly physical therapy? The initial assessment, the interventions, the revised plan of care are they truly being delivered by a licensed PT clinician or is he in effect delegating all aspects of care to an unlicensed person? And speaking about a license, George is only licensed in one jurisdiction, and does not have a compact privilege anywhere else. While the company said they make "every effort" to match him with people in the state he is licensed in …. He did not get the sense that they would turn away a client if he was not licensed in that state. For the **individual process** George is demonstrating moral sensitivity, recognizing that there is a potential ethical risk factor that he needs to have more information, before he can make an informed decision. George is comfortable with the idea that asking the right questions, he will avert a moral temptation.

Ethical Principles: The following principles guide his decision making,

3D: The physical therapist shall not engage in conflicts of interest that interfere with professional judgment.

8D: Physical therapists shall educate members of the public about the benefits of physical therapy and the unique role of the physical therapist. This principle includes guidance to carefully consider how people conceive of physical therapy and to be very careful that the impression the public has of the profession is accurate. If they receive substandard care that they think is PT, they and others may be easily dissuaded from trying PT again.

Ideas to Consider

1. Which is the least effective type of telehealth?
   a. Pure telehealth.
   b. Telecommunication.
   c. Hybrid telehealth.
   d. Artificial telehealth.

2. Telehealth is best described as which of the following?
   a. A type of treatment.
   b. A treatment modality.
   c. A location for treatment.
   d. A treatment decision.

3. Which of these does digital health include?
   a. Health care delivery technology.
   b. Wearable technology.
   c. a and b.
   d. Communication technology.

CHAPTER 8

Practicing a Hands-on Profession in a Hands-off World

Physical therapy is at its core a hands-on profession, It has become increasingly more challenging to practice safely and effectively when trust has been eroded by a few bad actors in health care who have made national headlines for sexual abuse. Our actions are guided by the foundation of the social contract between patient and clinician, Trust. In addition, regulations provide clear boundaries, and our professional behaviors are guided by our Code of Ethics and Standards of Ethical Conduct (Figure 8-1).

What is sexual misconduct and if you suspect it or see it …. What will you do about it?

Sexual misconduct is defined as:

1. Engaging in or soliciting sexual relationships, whether consensual or non-consensual, while a physical therapist or physical therapist assistant/patient relationship exists.
2. Making sexual advances, requesting sexual favors or engaging in other verbal conduct or physical contact of a sexual nature with patients or clients (MPA 6th Edition).

The Code of Ethics provides excellent guidance regarding sexual misconduct and harassment. 4E) Physical Therapists/Physical Therapist Assistants shall not engage in any sexual relationship with any of their patients and clients, supervisees, or students.

4F) Physical Therapists/Physical Therapist Assistants shall not harass anyone verbally, physically, emotionally, or sexually. Consult your practice act for explicit guidance. Most have some type of guidance regarding how long after the therapist patient relationship has ended before one can enter into a social relationship with a former patient. A word of caution here. As primary care providers for many patients the professional relationship is ongoing. We no longer talk about discharge but rather episodes of care that come to a conclusion recognizing that a new episode of care can begin at anytime.

As hands on practitioners, we always have to recognize that there is an increased vulnerability and chance that our actions may be misinterpreted, and we have to rely on excellent communication to make sure that the patient always understands what we are doing and why and is empowered to stop the interventions if they

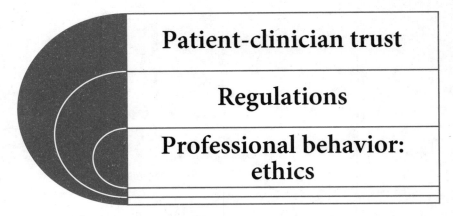

Figure 8-1 Foundation of professional behaviors

feel uncomfortable. True informed consent is critical here and it is important to remember that informed consent particularly for sensitive treatment is never sufficient if done just once when treatment commences. Informed consent is ongoing and modified as the treatment changes and progresses. The Code of Ethics provides clear guidance about this in **Principle 2C**: Physical therapists shall provide the information necessary to allow patients or their surrogates to make informed decisions about physical therapist care or participation in clinical research. The challenge is to leave no room for interpretation. Ask yourself the following questions throughout the patient contact. Where are your hands and how is that perceived? What is the intent of your hand placement and does the patient understand "the why?" Finally, how have you communicated your intentions and actions to the patient, do they understand and are they comfortable saying stop? It is not just about your hands; be careful of how you speak to the patient, how you look at them and be aware of the power of your body language.

While sexual misconduct is in the individual realm, we all know that the collateral damages from one clinician doing something inappropriate impacts the entire profession on the societal level (king, 2021, Lanier 2018, Morris, 2018) and may limit access for other patients who need physical therapy but have lost trust in the profession of physical therapy. Why are physical therapists more vulnerable than some of the other health care providers?

1. We tend to treat patients for a longer duration of time within an episode of care. This impacts the patient/therapist relationship.
2. We often treat in private, within an institution and home care. In this situation often patients are not fully clothed.
3. Our patients are vulnerable.

Sexual misconduct is a broad range of activities, from the seemingly innocuous word or gesture to truly egregious acts committed from a position of power. The Federation of State Boards of Medicine clearly defines these levels.

- Sexual Impropriety
  - Behaviors, gestures, expressions that are seductive, suggestive, disrespectful, or demeaning.
- Sexual Violation
  - Physical sexual conduct whether or not consented to by the patient.
- Sexual Assault
  - Sexual activity or contact without consent (physical force, threats of force, coercion, manipulation, imposition of power)
  - Law enforcement should be involved immediately.

The opportunity to become very aware of the sensitivities that individuals may have begins early in physical therapy education working with classmates and faculty, being sensitive to privacy and respect of the individual. This is the foundation of developing a culture of dignity and respect and patients should expect that regardless of treatment venue. We all recognize that there are certain societal norms and expectations but the standard for health care providers must be higher and in keeping with our Code of Ethics. Fortunately, the incidence of sexual misconduct among clinicians is low. However, we all recognize that just one inappropriate act can impact the profession as a whole so each of us has the responsibility to monitor our actions and the actions of our colleagues. The impact of sexual abuse on the individual is long-term (Starr, 2020). Recognizing the effects of sexual abuse is important to help people connect with the right provider and also to have a better understanding of how our actions may impact the patient. The classic effects of sexual abuse are found in Table 8-1.

Unfortunately, some abuse can take place with little accountability such as that found in social media. Social media is far reaching and permits the abuser anonymity and low accountability. It is far reaching with a long-term impact and a questionable true vs. not true factor.

PTs must be aware that patients they are seeing may come with preexisting trauma from a previous situation and may not share that information with the PT who is treating them. The PT must be vigilant in looking for signs such as reticence to provide information, or resistance to touch FSMB, 2020; Gallagher et al., 2021.

TABLE 8-1 EFFECTS OF SEXUAL ABUSE (DUBOIS ET AL., 2019)
Isolation
Confusion about role in the abuse
Loss of trust
Reluctance to seek help from another Health Care Provider
Anxiety/Panic
Depression
Sexual problems

To maintain credibility and trust professionals must take the responsibility to report inappropriate behavior and patients and family must be empowered to report actions that make them feel uncomfortable (Gallagher, 2021). Principle 4E provides clear guidance. "Physical therapists shall discourage misconduct by physical therapists, physical therapist assistants, and other health care professionals and, when appropriate, report illegal or unethical acts, including verbal, physical, emotional, or sexual harassment, to an appropriate authority with jurisdiction over the conduct." This is often difficult to do because the individual noting the potential abuse may be in a situation where the power is clearly not in their favor. Regarding the ethical responsibility of the PT in this type of situation we have to remember that the deliberate choice not to take action ... is in of itself an action (Bismark, 2020).

Not all actions of a sexual nature are initiated by the PT. Patients and patient's families have been noted in more than one situation to have initiated an inappropriate activity. Regardless of who initiates an activity the responsibility falls on the PT as they do have the power in the relationship and therefore the power to stop inappropriate actions. The power alone negates the chance for an equal consenting relationship.

PTs have to be vigilant and make sure that the relationship between the clinician and the patient/family remains professional. PTs constantly have to walk a narrow path between being friendly warm and welcoming to gain trust, and to being a friend which crosses a boundary. To decrease the risk of being accused of inappropriate behavior, it is important to keep the following in mind.

Consider using one or all three of the tools below to mitigate the risk of a sexual boundary crossing. Tools to mitigate the risk of a sexual boundary crossing.

Communication	Professional guidance	Take an ethical time out
Filter your speech. What you say How you say it Your body language	Use your Code of Ethics, and Standards of Ethical Conduct Know your practice act	Step back for a moment, time to think. What does it look like? Consult with a trusted other.

Case Study

Jack is an experienced home care therapist. He appreciates the opportunity to have direct patient care experiences and practice in such an independent primary care environment. He also enjoys interacting with the families and providing them with strategies that make working with their family members easier and more rewarding and empowering the entire family to manage the care. He arrives for his second visit with an elderly woman who is very debilitated. She lives with her husband Gus who is her caregiver. He was very reticent to answer many questions on the first visit. Jack noted that the home was very cluttered and the only place to really treat the patient was in her bed. He enters the bedroom and finds the patient on the bed completely naked with only a thin sheet near her. Jack turns to the husband as he leaves the room and asks him to please get his wife dressed for treatment. Gus responds, "she is more comfortable the way she is," and mumbles under his breath "I do enough for her. You want her dressed go right ahead. After all you are a Doctor what's the big deal?"

Recognize and Define the Ethical Issue

The situation is occurring in the individual realm between the therapist, patient, and caregiver. The individual process for Jack is initially moral sensitivity, taking the time to reflect on how his actions may appear and being sensitive to the rights of the patient but also protecting himself from a potential situation in which he may be wrongly accused of inappropriate behavior. Jack is faced with an ethical problem, a threat to his moral duties and values.

Reflect

In addition to the issues facing Jack about establishing an appropriate treatment environment, he is also concerned about the relationship between the patient and caregiver. While not necessarily suspecting abuse Gus seems overwhelmed, and he may benefit from some social service intervention.

The following principles from the Code of Ethics guide Jack in his decision-making.

2D: Physical therapists shall collaborate with patients/clients to empower them in decisions about their healthcare.

3A: Physical therapists shall demonstrate independent and objective professional judgment in the patient's/client's best interest in all practice settings.

3C: Physical therapists shall make judgments within their scope of practice and level of expertise and shall communicate with, collaborate with or refer to peers or other healthcare professionals when necessary.

CHAPTER 9

The Ethical Challenges of the Future

Ethical decision-making evolves as healthcare evolves. The choices that we have expand, but the basic parameters by which we make these changes are a constant, providing a frame of reference and stability in an exciting and ever-evolving healthcare landscape.

Consider for example end-of-life issues. When medicine had no options to offer, there were few ethical choices to make. As medicine progressed and there were options available to keep people alive, we were faced with the ethical questions of not only whether we should keep people alive but how and when we should allow people to die.

For every improvement in healthcare, there are hopefully concurrent improvements in quality of life, which of course is an area that physical therapists become actively engaged in. The exciting thing about this topic is that as quickly as new technology is introduced it is outdated with the next breakthrough in the wings ready to take its place. The challenge for us as healthcare providers is to choose wisely when embracing new techniques and technology. Rehabilitation is considered the downstream recipient of new developments as we translate the advancements into function. We are still concerned with the same issues, such as fairness in access, and justice in resource allocation. We have to be mindful that we don't expend more time and resources on a patient or technology just because of the novelty of a new process or intervention. Technology also demands of us responsible research and responsible care.

Between the first edition of this book and this publication the topics that follow have continued to evolve and some have become mainstream practice By no means is this a complete listing either; it is meant to be a start, a jumping off point for you to begin to think of the many other things that while in development should be considered as to their impact on the delivery of physical therapy and the future of physical therapy treatment. To fully assess the value of new techniques and technology, the patient must remain the central focus. Each new technique or technology must be evaluated based on its risk–benefit ratio, its worth, a function of cost and value, and the possible positive and negative consequences.

New techniques in physical therapy Access and allocation
Genomics and gene therapy
Therapeutic procedures in utero Stem cell therapy

Consideration of non-opioid treatment options Using exercise with serious illnesses
Telehealth and digital PT care at a distance see the chapter dedicated to this area.
Robotics
Artificial Intelligence

New Techniques in Physical Therapy:
New techniques in physical therapy are constantly evolving. PTs have an ethical obligation to remain current with changes in the field. Principle **6:** "Physical therapists shall enhance their expertise through the lifelong acquisition and refinement of knowledge, skills, abilities, and professional behaviors." PTs also have the obligation to evaluate new techniques and determine the value of that technique for their practice. Principle **6C:** "Physical therapists shall evaluate the strength of evidence and applicability of content presented during professional development activities before integrating the content or techniques into practice." The other challenge that physical therapists have to keep in mind when integrating new techniques and technology is the techniques are applied to those who will benefit from them and as much as possible the techniques are available to the population that needs them. Principle **8B:** "Physical therapists shall advocate to reduce health disparities and healthcare inequities, approve access to healthcare services, and address the health, wellness, and preventive healthcare needs of people."

Genomics and Gene Therapy:
Exciting research into the world of personalized medicine characterizes genomics and gene therapy. Diseases such as cystic fibrosis and sickle cell anemia caused by a single defective gene can be treated before symptoms become severe as a child's genome can be sequenced at birth. There is transformative potential in gene therapy and the resulting challenges and opportunities to help patients achieve a high quality of life fall squarely in the world of the physical therapist. What cannot be ignored in the world of genomics is the impact that the ability to modify the genome can mean from the perspective of "a designer or designed population." This is a classic example of the ethical imperative to consider, "just because we can, does it mean we should?" We have to carefully consider the options that technology permits. The ability of the scientific community to alter genomes leads to the opportunity to create "designer babies" with the potential for the creation of the perfect human race. The ethical implications are challenging (Juengst et al., 2016).

Therapeutic Procedures in Utero:
The ability to influence a potentially negative outcome at birth by interventions in utero can have significant impact on financial resources as well as healthcare and education resources. The most significant impact is of course the individual whose quality of life can be significantly altered. The identification of defects and repair of the same in utero could have a significant impact on the types of patient's physical therapists see in the future. The number of future patients could also change as more babies survive and thrive past their first birthday. Others may not need the extensive level

of care that they would have had without the in utero intervention which permitted them to survive (Wojcicki and Drozdowski, 2010). The impact on the survival rate and the quality of life for all involved with a multiple birth is significant. Growth and development are easily monitored and where possible therapeutic interventions implemented early in the pregnancy to help carry multiple babies to term.

Stem Cell Research:
Some of the most promising and innovative research in the late 20th- and early 21st-century has to do with stem cell research and the implications it has for quality of life for people with a myriad of medical problems such as spinal cord injuries and chronic diseases. Similar to the innovations in genomics and in utero procedures, the many benefits of the application of the stem cell line of inquiry must be carefully weighed vs. the concerns about this new frontier in healthcare. The medical breakthroughs are more than promising, but the business ventures supporting the line of inquiry must be held to the highest standard to ensure that the research is about what benefits patients, without undue harm (Hagan, 2013).

Non-Opioid Treatment Options to Reduce Pain:
Consideration of non-opioid treatment options is a very popular topic currently, and yet pain reduction using PT therapeutic treatment options has been a part of physical therapy since the inception of the field. So, what is the ethical imperative here? This is a great example of the importance placed on the societal responsibility that physical therapists have to validate what physical therapy can do, and then to help the public and the medical community recognize the value of PT (Taylor, 2017), Principle 8D: "Physical therapists shall educate members of the public about the benefits of physical therapy and the unique role of the physical therapist" It is the responsibility of the professional community to disseminate information that can be of value. In an effort to address pain physical therapists are appearing more regularly in the emergency department of the hospital, providing patients with postural modifications, work saving techniques and options for non-narcotic pain relief in collaboration with other members of the health care team such as physicians and pharmacists (Gagnon, 2021; Kim, 2021; Mourad et al., 2022; Strudwick et al., 2022).

Using Exercise with Serious Illness:
Individuals with complex medical conditions often were cautioned against exercise, and this lack of mobility often increased morbidity. This is an example of an evolving treatment rationale that is a mainstream recommendation in most situations, with very clear-cut treatment advantages (Shih et al., 2015). Once again, collecting relevant evidence and sharing that evidence with the public and the medical community changes the norms and adjusts the expected outcomes. The Code of Ethics encourages the PT to share information.

"Principle 2C: Physical therapists shall provide the information necessary to allow patients or their surrogates to make informed decisions about physical therapy care or participation in clinical research."

Robotics:

The technical advantages of robotics are in the research and innovation stage. For PTs, as for other healthcare providers, the ethical issues with robotics center around the relationship between the provider and the patient. The use of robotics is similar to using any other type of technology as an adjunct to care. Consistent with any research endeavor, actions should be guided by responsible research requirements. The functional use of robotics in rehabilitation to improve quality of life for patients is in the nascent exploratory stages. Biomedical engineering coupled with physical therapy expertise is a natural alliance (Stahl and Coeckelbergh, 2016).

Regardless of the innovation the physical therapist may choose to use to enhance patient care, keeping the patient as the central focus ensures that these encounters benefit from appropriate ethical guidance.

Artificial Intelligence:

Access to big data has made some of the PT processes amenable to the application of Artifical Intelligence to some clinical tasks. PTs are encouraged to see where AI may be of benefit to improve access and to improve outcomes. AI applications have the potential to have a very positive impact on outcomes but for widespread use to be feasible PT's must become familiar with AI and how it may be applied to their practice setting including the potential risks and benefits (Mashael, 2022).

PART TWO

Types of Ethical Decisions: Case Analysis

CHAPTER 10

Introduction to Case Analysis

Unless otherwise noted, cases were previously published in PT in Motion and APTA Magazine, and are adapted with permission from the American Physical Therapy Association

The next section of this book consists of case commentaries and opportunities for discussion. The most effective way to incorporate ethical decision-making into clinical practice is to have the opportunity to have case discussions. This section allows you to use these case discussions in a variety of ways.

They can be discussed in a large group, or the elements of the ethical decision-making process can be analyzed individually and then discussed in a variety of types of feedback sessions.

Regardless of how the cases are utilized they are arranged to provide the PT, PTA, and students with opportunities to develop clinical ethical decision-making skills that complement their clinical decision-making abilities.

There are eight case sections in this portion of the book. Cases are placed in the appropriate section to demonstrate the wide variety of ethical issues that confront practitioners. There is of course considerable overlap between the cases and the issues that they portray. Discussing multiple cases in a section can reinforce the fact that often a similar type of issue will present itself very differently, but a clinician using an organized form of analysis will recognize common features to help them manage the specific situation before them. At the end of each case, there is a section entitled *Consider and Reflect*; this allows the reader an opportunity to look into the thought processes of the primary stakeholders. Examining the situation from the perspective of the main characters may help frame your ethical decision-making.

There are many ways in which your opinion may differ from other clinicians, and you may have a very different take on the situation you are encouraged to provide that. However, it is important that you always approach an ethical decision using an ethical decision-making process. Initially this may seem a bit "clunky," but it will become part of your systematic thinking just as the structure of a patient evaluation becomes natural and fluid.

There is one other thing to keep in mind when developing an ethical response. Resolution of one issue may result in an adverse effect for some stakeholders, and it is important to keep the idea of "collateral damages" in mind and weigh whether or not the actions decided upon are worth the potential problems.

This introduction starts with a fully developed case, to provide guidance into one way in which this case can be analyzed. There are many ways in which to analyze an ethical issue, but what they have in common is a systematic approach that provides the clinician with common factors that are easily referred to in future analysis. As clinical experience develops so should all of the professional behaviors that include the ethical foundations for clinical practice.

Use the example that follows: *It's not in my job description* to enhance your understanding of the ethical decision-making process. Script font in the Ethical Decision-Making Worksheet indicates student answers. Subsequent cases will allow you to develop your own reasoning and justifications for your decisions.

The following case is an example of how to review a case and analyze it using a modified version of the RIPS model.

Case Example 1

IT'S NOT IN MY JOB DESCRIPTION!

The clinical portion of professional education is managed differently in different fields. For example, our colleagues in nursing are generally accompanied into the clinical setting with dedicated academic faculty who continue the didactic instruction in the clinical setting. The staff nurses in the setting, though available for consultation, are primarily dedicated to patient care. Our colleagues in occupational therapy have a model of clinical education that is similar to what we have in physical therapy. In both disciplines, the clinical aspect of the education is performed off-site, and the instructors are clinicians. As programs enlarge class sizes and new programs emerge the competition for clinical sites becomes even more of a challenge.

Bruce chose his position at The Rehab Institute (TRI) very carefully a year ago when he graduated. It had all of his "must haves" in a position, and now just a short year later as he reflected on all the experiences he had had, he confirmed what a great choice he had made. At his annual review, he discussed the next steps with his supervisor Shelly. He arranged to stay on the Neuro floor for another rotation because he was starting his preparation for the Neurological Clinical Specialist exam. He was promoted from Staff PT to lead PT assigned to the Neuro I gym. Bruce was obviously very excited about the new opportunities for him to grow professionally. Of all the things that he and Shelly discussed, the one that excited him, but scared him, the most was the new status earned by his longevity at The Rehab Institute, he was now a *Clinical Instructor*. In just four weeks, he was going to be working with his first student. While he was excited about the opportunity to share this exciting clinical experience with a future colleague, he could not help but question how ready he was to guide somebody, just one year his junior, through the complex world of clinical practice. Shelly also shared with Bruce that the Neuro I gym has become an area in the hospital where few students could rotate because not many of the clinicians were willing to take students. She encouraged him to make that a priority; she really wanted to be able to offer more rotations in this area. Bruce didn't bring it up with Shelly, but he was a bit confused. He never thought that it was an option whether or not you had a student. The Rehab Institute was a large teaching facility world renowned for patient care and student training in a host of disciplines. One of the reasons he came here was for the opportunity to participate in a strong student clinical education program, he just assumed it was one of the attractions to everybody who came to work at TRI. Bruce quickly sought out his mentor Lynn who was on the post-surgical floor to get her take on the charge Shelly gave Bruce. She concurred with Shelly that few of the therapists on Neuro I were willing to take students citing a variety of reasons, but primarily the workload, and the acuity of the patients on that floor making a student experience somewhat complicated. Bruce was still not convinced, thinking there had to be other reasons, conflicting vacation schedules, incompatible rotation times with the assigned students, certainly the cause was something that could be administratively corrected. He was determined to get to the cause and as his first contribution to TRI in a position of more responsibility he was going to make sure that Neuro I was one of the most productive clinical education sites in the entire hospital. He sought out the other seven team members from Neuro I and quickly realized that four of them had not had a student in over two years and one had never had a student. The remaining two therapists had two students during the past year and when questioned by Bruce quickly responded that they were "burnt out" tired, and really wanted to concentrate on their own patients for a little while. Bruce had never been in that position, so he accepted their word, confident that they would return to the rotation within the year. He focused on the five therapists who have not recently had students and was given quite an earful. Their comments ranged from "no reason to put out all the effort a student requires" to "students these days are too demanding," and one that was particularly baffling "students distract me from providing good patient care." They were not the answers Bruce expected from his colleagues. Bruce always thought that having a student would stimulate you to constantly reflect on how and why you were doing something. Bruce had never given it very much thought before, but if PTs and PTAs were unwilling to supervise students what would happen to professional education? Wasn't the responsibility to "pay it forward" a professional obligation? He was not sure that this was going to be as easy a fix as he thought, his colleagues did not seem to be very invested in the idea of clinical education as part of insuring their own professional growth and continuing competence. Bruce was amazed; he thought that when you take a job in a place like TRI, it is with the implicit understanding that you will supervise students. Bruce felt strongly that participation in clinical education should not be optional. He was determined to find guidance from the core documents supporting participation in the clinical education of the students.

CONSIDER AND REFLECT

The unique partnership in education between the didactic learning received at the University and the clinical education received in a practice setting has been the longstanding accepted norm for physical therapy. Whether the often-touted benefits of professional development and recruitment outweigh the perceived increase to workload is subject to debate, but central to this question is the professional responsibility to educate the next generation of clinicians. Not all facilities nor all clinicians are up to the task, should it be expected as part of practice or remain just those who self-identify with the interest and the ability to provide a positive clinical experience? Should there be an expectation that every PT is capable of guiding a student through a clinical experience and it should be the minimum expected for clinical competence? If clinical education is spread across more clinicians wouldn't that decrease the workload on just a few and eliminate the burnout while potentially raising the practice standard for those that have avoided clinical education because of concerns of their own abilities and competencies?

Bruce is surprised that what he considers to be the norm in good practice and professional behavior is not interpreted that way by all. Can a facility mandate participation in clinical education when it is not direct patient care, the primary reason the clinician was hired? What is his professional responsibility?

After working through the ethical decision-making process, what course of action would you suggest?

Ethical Decision-Making Worksheet

Case: *It's not in my job description*

The Realm   Jack Glaser (1994)

Individual	Organizational/ Institutional	Societal
The good of the patient/ client and focuses on rights, duties, relationships, and behaviors between individuals	Good of the organization, focuses on structures and systems, which facilitate organizational or institutional goals	Concerned with the common good

The Realm: *Organizational/Institutional*

Rationale: *Some facilities see clinical education as both a philosophical and a practical mandate. Philosophically, providing good clinical experiences is the right thing to do. Practically, it is a good staff motivator to strive for excellence and not a bad recruitment tool.*

The Individual Process

James Rest (1994, 1999)

Moral Sensitivity	Moral Judgment	Moral Motivation	Moral Courage	Moral Potency (Hannah and Avolio, 2010)
Recognizing, interpreting, and framing an ethical situation	Right vs. wrong actions. Generating options, selecting and applying ethical principles	Priority on ethical values over other values. Professionalism is a primary motivator for ethical behavior	Implementing the chosen ethical action, development of a plan	Includes decision making that includes moral ownership, courage and self-efficacy

The Individual Process: *Moral sensitivity*

Rationale: *Bruce sees the responsibility of working with students as an ethical issue, part of his professional responsibility.*

The Situation

Swisher et al. (2005) adapted from Kidder

Issue/ Problem	Dilemma	Distress	Temptation	Silence
Important values present	Two alternative courses of action: Right vs. Right decision	The right course of action is known but the clinician cannot perform it	Choice between right and wrong	Values are challenged but no one is speaking about this challenge to values

The Situation: *Ethical issue/problem*

Rationale: *The value of excellence is central to professional behaviors consistent with professional engagement.*

Ethical Principles and/or Standards of Ethical Conduct of the PTA

Code of Ethics (Principles) for PTs	Rationale	Standards of Ethical Conduct (Standards) for PTAs	Rationale
Principle 6D: Physical therapists shall cultivate practice environments that support professional development, lifelong learning, and excellence	Professional development includes lifelong learning and excellence		

(continued on following page)

Suggested Action: *Approaching a local education institution to provide information about the advantage of being engaged in clinical education and how the institution can provide support to encourage clinical education involvement.*

CHAPTER 11

Accountability

All healthcare professionals are expected to be accountable. Physical therapists and physical therapist assistants are of course no exception—accountability is one of the virtues that is a core value of the profession. The confusion that occurs regarding accountability centers on who the PT/PTA is accountable to, because in many cases there may be multiple equally compelling demands on the PT/PTA. At all times the first and primary demand for accountability is a result of the patient/therapist relationship. It is always important to keep this relationship in mind through all interactions, as it is the foundation of the ethical and clinical decision making that physical therapists engage in. Of course, it would be simple if that were the only party that the PT/PTA was accountable to, but there are many. The PT/PTA also has to be accountable to the organization that they work within, whether employed, contracted, or self-employed. In addition, the PT/PTA has a responsibility to the profession. How do the actions of the PT/PTA impact the profession as a whole? How is each PT/PTA accountable to maintaining the reputation of physical therapy and helping physical therapy to continue to grow and develop? There is also accountability to society. How will our actions impact things like access to care and promotion of health and wellness? No less important is the accountability the physical therapist/assistant must have to themselves. A PT/PTA is more vulnerable to poor ethical and clinical decisions when his or her own well-being is compromised, and the PT/PTA must take the responsibility to recognize his or her own vulnerability. Accountability is complex and integral to fulfilling our responsibilities to our patients, fully cognizant that we do not practice in isolation we are part of a healthcare team and organization with responsibilities to society. In the cases that follow, we will look at accountability from several different vantage points.

Destination Dilemma — Best interest determination
What Happens In Pt, Stays In Pt — Patient confidentiality vs. professional duty
Sticks and Stones — Patient–therapist relationship challenges
All that is new and shiny — Who stands to benefit?

Case Example 1

DESTINATION DILEMMA
Best interest determination

Physical therapists (PTs) in the acute care setting are expected not only to be excellent care providers, but also to provide the healthcare team with

87

expert guidance on whether and in what setting additional care is appropriate. There are factors, however, that can cloud the issue of where the patient goes next. Consider the following scenario.

Brad is a PT at an acute care hospital. He finds the practice setting challenging but deeply gratifying, as he plays an important role in improving the condition of patients who are recovering from significant debilitation due to illness or injury.

Patients and their families rely on Brad's guidance as post-discharge options are weighed. In which setting will the family member do best? Long-term acute care? A subacute facility? Acute rehab? Home care? Brad takes pride in his ability to walk patients and families through an unfamiliar maze of terms and options. He is good at explaining that, while three hours a day of rehabilitation might seem like the quickest route to recovery, the patient may not be able to safely tolerate that. Often, Brad points out, placing the patient in a less-intensive environment produces the same long-term results; it just takes more time.

Brad is well aware, however, that, in some cases, the degree of a patient's progress may make him or her ineligible for the level of care he deems most appropriate. He is adept at what he calls "managing the system"—meticulously documenting and carefully planning interventions in such a way as to optimally prepare the patient for safe discharge to the correct level of care. He is committed to effectively advocating for his patients while playing by the rules.

He knows of PTs, however, who have, for example, been instructed by their supervisor to "tweak" documentation to help get a patient accepted into acute rehab. He's heard of circumstances, too, in which PTs have been told to follow a documentation template to meet patient-admission criteria for an extended care facility. Many PTs, Brad realizes, are under increasing pressure to get patients placed quickly into settings that serve to improve hospitals' length-of-stay statistics. Brad fortunately has not faced any such situations.

The case of Donald puts Brad in an uncomfortable position. Donald is a 64-year-old man who had a stroke that produced mild left hemiparesis. His motor function has improved significantly, but he has significant perceptual losses. Brad considers Donald to be an unsafe ambulator without close supervision, and thus recommends a period of inpatient rehabilitation.

Donald's "shared risk" healthcare insurance will not, however, cover all the expenses of an inpatient stay. His physician and the care coordinator say that they feel he will be fine at home. Donald is inclined to trust their judgment and save out-of-pocket costs.

Having completed a fall risk assessment based on Donald's home floor plan, current medications, and Berg and Tinetti balance results, Brad is deeply concerned that his patient is at significant fall risk, and that returning him to his home increases the chance that he will sustain a fracture, resulting in greater disability. Brad shares his findings and concerns with Donald and his family, but they are convinced having seen remarkable improvement in motor function that the perceptual and cognitive issues will clear just as fast.

Brad knows, though, that if he documents in great detail his findings and recommendations, he will be placing the hospital at greater liability risk should Donald be released to home care, fall there, and sustain further injury. On the other hand, Brad reasons, perhaps such detailed documentation will convince Donald's physician and care coordinator to reconsider their plan to send the patient home and instead will authorize inpatient rehabilitation. Brad is aware that inpatient care may be more expensive initially, but the long-term result should be significantly better requiring Donald to need less care overall and therefore almost neutralize the initial higher expense. He is not convinced that the family, based on his previous conversation, would be very accepting of the rationale for this plan. Donald considers his options about how to proceed.

REFLECT

Brad must decide whether or not to document in detail the extent of Donald's fall risk. One option would expose the hospital to a type of risk, while the other would expose Donald to a different type of risk. Based on his experience and professional judgment, Brad feels that Donald would benefit from a course of inpatient rehabilitation. Brad's non-rehab colleagues at the hospital, however, advocate for home care. Donald is fine with that as he is concerned about the out-of-pocket expense he may incur. What is his colleagues' motivation? Brad wonders. Professional judgment? Institutional concerns? Appreciation of the patient's pocketbook issues? Some combination thereof? Brad has to consider his own motivation and make sure that he is considering all perspectives and desires ....

After working through the ethical decision-making process, what course of action would you suggest?

Ethical Decision-Making Worksheet

Case: _____

The Realm   Jack Glaser (1994)

Individual	Organizational/ Institutional	Societal
The good of the patient/client and focuses on rights, duties, relationships and behaviors between individuals	Good of the organization, focuses on structures and systems, which facilitate organizational or institutional goals	Concerned with the common good

(continued on following page)

The Realm _____

Rationale:

The Individual Process: James Rest (1994, 1999)

Moral Sensitivity	Moral Judgment	Moral Motivation	Moral Courage	Moral Potency (Hannah and Avolio, 2010)
Recognizing, interpreting, and framing an ethical situation	Right versus wrong actions. Generating options, selecting and applying ethical principles	Priority on ethical values over other values. Professionalism is a primary motivator for ethical behavior	Implementing the chosen ethical action, development of a plan	Includes decision making that includes moral ownership, courage, and self-efficacy

The Individual Process: _____

Rationale:

The Situation   Swisher et al. (2005) adapted from Kidder

Issue/ Problem	Dilemma	Distress	Temptation	Silence
Important values present	Two alternative courses of action: Right vs. Right decision	The right course of action is known but the clinician cannot perform it	Choice between right and wrong	Values are challenged but no one is speaking about this challenge to values

The Situation: _____

Rationale: _____

_____

Ethical Principles and/or Standards of Ethical Conduct of the PTA (see Appendixes A and B)

(continued on following page)

Code of Ethics (Principles) for PTs	Rationale	Standards of Ethical Conduct (Standards) for PTAs	Rationale

Suggested Action:

Case Example 2

WHAT HAPPENS IN PT, STAYS IN PT
Patient confidentiality vs. professional duty

Principle 2 of the Code of Ethics for Physical Therapist states, "Physical therapists shall be trustworthy and compassionate in addressing the rights and needs of patients/clients." The statement is straightforward, but its manifestations and ramifications are not simple. Consider the following case of a parent who feels betrayed and a physical therapist (PT) who questions his own actions.

Ben is a board-certified specialist in pediatric physical therapy at Rocking Ridge Children's Services. He has enjoyed his ten years there serving children and their families.

Among his patients is Andy, who is almost five years old and has significant mobility limitations and impaired perception. Ben has been working with Judy, Andy's mother, to ensure Andy's safety as well as his optimal mobility. Judy has been a dedicated advocate for her son, but she also has a daughter who is almost four and six-week-old twin boys. At times she says things like, "Four kids under 5 years old! What was I thinking?" and "This menagerie will kill me yet!" with exasperated humor.

When Judy's mother, Beatrice, brings Andy in for four straight appointments, Ben worries, because Andy's progress has concurrently regressed. Ben feels that Judy's hands-on presence is important to her son's care. He is relieved, therefore, when Judy arrives with Andy for the next appointment. But she has brought her other children with her as well, explaining that her mother has flown west to scout out an assisted living facility near the home of her son Paul, Judy's brother.

Although Ben well-appreciates the multiple pressures parents face, and has great patience with multitasking moms and dads and rambunctious children, the therapy visit with Judy and her four children quickly becomes challenging. Amy, the lone daughter, is running around the room. The twins are crying. Judy is distracted as Ben tries to talk with her. Andy is fidgeting as if distressed by all the commotion. Judy clearly is harried. Ben tries to put her at ease, saying, "I remember when my kids were young. They can be a handful, can't they?"

Judy smiles weakly and says, "Soon I won't have mom to help me out. I don't know what I'm going to do."

Ben tries to be supportive. "You always find a way," he says. "You got Andy through his early-intervention years and have really helped his development. Your children are lucky to have you as their mom. Maybe your husband can spell you a bit more often? Anyway, before you know it, Amy will be in school. That will take some pressure off."

"I just don't know anymore," Judy responds dolefully. She smooths Andy's hair, stares for several seconds at Ben's diploma on the wall, then suddenly blurts out, "I just don't know how much longer I can do this! Sometimes I feel like I'm losing it. I get so frustrated! I've never laid a hand on my kids in anger, but some days I feel like I could really hurt 1 of them, when it all seems like too much."

Ben is stunned. He appreciates the fact that parents can feel overwhelmed. He has felt that himself at times. But this seems like a different level of distress. Is it just Judy's fatigue talking, or is it a real cry for help?

The session ends on a calmer note, with the babies pacified, Amy leafing through picture books, and Ben and Judy able to focus on Andy and his needs. Judy even says before she leaves, "Please forget about that thing I said before. You're right. I'll be fine."

But Ben cannot forget about it. Later that morning, he calls Beth, Andy's referring pediatrician. He recounts the conversation with Judy and asks Beth what she thinks. "This *is* a post-partum mother we're talking about," Ben observes. "Maybe this sort of thing gets said sometimes, and it's an isolated comment and isn't necessarily a red flag. Should I—should we—be concerned?"

There's a long pause on the other end of the line. "Judy's never said anything like that to me," Beth finally responds.

"Well, what, if anything, should I do about it?" Ben asks.

"It's a tough call, I'll grant you," Beth says. But she declines to advise him further. She thanks him for the call and says that she has a patient to see.

Ben wishes Beth had given him clear guidance. But he, too, gets on with his day, resolving to give the matter more thought that evening. Just as he's preparing to leave the office later that afternoon, however, he gets a phone call from Judy. She is furious.

"It can't be a coincidence that I told you something in confidence this morning that I didn't really mean, and that just hours later Social Services was at my door!" Judy fumes. "Now I've got a case file and have been told that I can expect observation visits. Thanks a lot! It looks like I'm in the market for a new PT—someone I can trust!" With that, she hangs up.

For the second time that day, Ben is stunned. He had no inkling Beth would call Social Services after he had spoken with her. While he might have ended up calling the agency himself, he also might have decided against it—or at least might have waited to see if Judy would repeat her disturbing comments on a future visit.

He now wonders whether he erred in calling Beth. Had he overstepped? Had he actually caused harm in his attempt to prevent it?

CONSIDER AND REFLECT

Ben feels that some type of action is necessary, and he determines that it's best to discuss the matter with Andy's pediatrician as a first step.

Diagnosing a patient or caregiver/guardian's mental health is outside of Ben's scope of practice, but he is sufficiently disturbed by Judy's words that he feels he must share them with the referring physician. While the PT makes clear that he is simply seeking the physician's opinion, his doing so causes a chain of events that deeply upsets Judy, and places her under intense scrutiny. Do you think Ben acted appropriately? How would you have responded to Judy's outburst? In making every effort to be accountable how was it perceived by the patient's family and what does it represent in the relationship between the two healthcare providers.

After working through the ethical decision-making process, what course of action would you suggest?

Ethical Decision-Making Worksheet

Case: _____

The Realm: Jack Glaser (1994)

Individual	Organizational/ Institutional	Societal
The good of the patient/client and focuses on rights, duties, relationships, and behaviors between individuals	Good of the organization, focuses on structures and systems, which facilitate organizational or institutional goals	Concerned with the common good

The Realm: _____

Rationale:

The Individual Process: James Rest (1994, 1999)

Moral Sensitivity	Moral Judgment	Moral Motivation	Moral Courage	Moral Potency (Hannah and Avolio, 2010)
Recognizing, interpreting, and framing an ethical situation	Right vs. wrong actions. Generating options, selecting and applying ethical principles	Priority on ethical values over other values. Professionalism is a primary motivator for ethical behavior	Implementing the chosen ethical action, development of a plan	Includes decision making that includes moral ownership, courage, and self-efficacy

The Individual Process: _____

Rationale:

The Situation: Swisher et al. (2005) adapted from Kidder

Issue/ Problem	Dilemma	Distress	Temptation	Silence
Important values present	Two alternative courses of action: Right vs. Right decision	The right course of action is known but the clinician cannot perform it	Choice between right and wrong	Values are challenged but no one is speaking about this challenge to values

(continued on following page)

The Situation: _____

Rationale:

Ethical Principles and/or Standards of Ethical Conduct of the PTA (see Appendixes A and B)

Code of Ethics (Principles) for PTs	Rationale	Standards of Ethical Conduct (Standards) for PTAs	Rationale

Suggested Action:

Case Example 3

STICKS AND STONES
Patient–therapist relationship challenges

Physical therapists (PTs) and physical therapist assistants understand that patients who have certain diagnoses and conditions may have secondary behavioral issues. They are trained to manage the situation in the manner that best serves and respects the rights of all parties, including other patients and clients. What is their responsibility, however, when there is no apparent health-related reason for inappropriate patient language or actions? How much should a healthcare provider reasonably be expected to take?

As a certified neurology specialist (NSC), Diane leads patients—many of them senior citizens—through her hospital's balance training system.

It is deeply gratifying work, helping to restore the confidence and physical stability of individuals whose balance issues are significant and whose fear of falling is acute. She relishes the atmosphere of mutual trust she builds with her patients.

Returning to her floor after lunch one afternoon, Diane is surprised to hear a male voice profanely shouting in the distance. She is scheduled to see a new patient, Frank, a 54-year-old man with multiple sclerosis (MS), but that is not a condition that is known to provoke aggression or impropriety. Surely the string of expletives Diane is hearing couldn't be issuing from her new patient's mouth?

When she reaches the waiting area, however, the first words she hears are, "Well, well, well. I'm Frank Greenleigh, and, let me guess, you're the physical therapist who's been keeping me waiting. It's about [censored] time!"

Taken aback, Diane glances at the clock on the wall, which confirms that it is exactly 1:00 pm, Frank's appointment time. Cheryl, the receptionist, volunteers, "Mr. Greenleigh, um, arrived a bit early today."

Frank responds by shouting, while pointing at Diane, "I wasn't early! You were late!"

Diane responds in a calm and measured voice, "The important thing is, I'm here now. Let's go through that door to your right, and I'll show you where I can have a look at you." Frank scowls and makes grumbling sounds, but he says nothing further as he accompanies Diane into an examination room.

Frank is grudgingly cooperative during Diane's evaluation and initial interventions. But then, when he experiences discomfort while completing a task, he shouts in a voice loud enough to be heard several rooms away, "You [censored]! What the [censored] are you trying to do to me here? I already have MS! Isn't that enough [censored] for me to have to deal with?"

Stunned by the outburst, Diane takes a deep breath, then says, "Mr. Greenleigh, I had informed you that some discomfort was likely, but please tell me what you're feeling, and we'll try to make adjustments along the way. OK? That kind of language really isn't called for."

A wide smile spreads across Frank's face. "Aw, can't you tell when I'm just playing with you?" he asks. "I'm guessing you've never been in the service, or spent much time around old Army cusses like me. Why don't you try to relax! You people are a little uptight."

Diane responds with a sigh, "I have the utmost respect for those who serve our country, but profane and disrespectful language is uncalled for and upsetting to everyone here, including our other patients and staff. Whether you're kidding or not, I must again ask you to watch your language and be mindful of where you are."

"Hey, the last time I looked, I was in America, where we have this little constitutional right called freedom of speech," Frank says heatedly. "Now, how about, instead of reading me the riot act, you do your job—preferably without torturing me—and we get on with this, you [censored]?" He then grins slightly, as if to say his fury isn't to be taken entirely seriously.

Diane defers to Frank for the rest of his visit. He does not shout again or issue any other profanities, but he does alternate between taking inappropriate umbrage and offering conciliatory assurances that he is "just joking around."

Meanwhile, Diane is formulating a plan: Before his next appointment, she will get Frank switched to the hospital across town, where he will pair up with her no-nonsense colleague Jim. He is an ex-marine who, like Diane, is an NSC experienced in leading patients through balance training.

Once Frank has left the hospital, Diane presents her plan to Dan, her immediate supervisor. "I understand what you're saying," he says. "I was behind a closed door and I still heard that outburst in the reception area. He's a piece of work. You do realize, though, that I'll need to run this by Cathy."

Later that afternoon, after Diane has completed a visit with another patient, Cathy—the "big boss"—walks over and says, "Listen, I appreciate the discomfort you felt. But you can't just discharge Mr. Greenleigh to someone else's care. He's your patient. You and he have started a relationship, even if it had a rocky start. If you just send him on his way, it's abandonment. And that doesn't wash. Sorry."

As Cathy walks away, Diane looks on with disappointment and surprise. Where is it written that she must simply take Frank's abuse? Is Cathy's veto the last word? What are the ethics and legalities here? Doesn't Diane have rights in this situation?

CONSIDER AND REFLECT

Legally speaking, Principle 5A is the place to start. Laws regarding patient discharge and abandonment are jurisdiction-specific and governed by state practice acts. Diane would be well advised to consult hers. In addition, principle 5F speaks specifically to the transfer of care and how it is accomplished without abandoning the patient.

PTs are responsible to make every effort to meet patients and clients "where they are" and to help them benefit, to the greatest extent possible, from the expertise offered by the PT. It is also reasonable to conclude that a PT who feels uncomfortable or threatened may not be an optimally effective practitioner. There are the needs and rights of others within the hospital environment to consider in this case, as well. How might Diane best reconcile these differences in a way that is fair to all parties?

Diane has seen Mr. Greenleigh only once. Mightn't things get better? Should the fact that there is no apparent medical rationale for Frank's behavior be a consideration one way or the other?

Yet, one could argue, mightn't Diane, hospital staff, other patients, and Frank himself be better served by placing him under the care of a PT who might be better able to modify his behavior? Isn't it possible that Frank, in fact, will respect and defer to a fellow veteran?

What does the Code of Ethics for the Physical Therapist have to say in support or rejection of Diane's desire to discharge Frank?

After working through the ethical decision-making process, what course of action would you suggest?

Ethical Decision-Making Worksheet

Case: _____

The Realm   Jack Glaser (1994)

Individual	Organizational/ Institutional	Societal
The good of the patient/client and focuses on rights, duties, relationships, and behaviors between individuals	Good of the organization, focuses on structures and systems, which facilitate organizational or institutional goals	Concerned with the common good

The Realm: _____

Rationale:

The Individual Process: James Rest (1994, 1999)

Moral Sensitivity	Moral Judgment	Moral Motivation	Moral Courage	Moral Potency (Hannah and Avolio, 2010)
Recognizing, interpreting, and framing an ethical situation	Right vs. wrong actions. Generating options, selecting, and applying ethical principles	Priority on ethical values over other values. Professionalism is a primary motivator for ethical behavior	Implementing the chosen ethical action, development of a plan	Includes decision making that includes moral ownership, courage, and self-efficacy

(continued on following page)

The Individual Process: _____

Rationale:

The Situation   Swisher et al. (2005) adapted from Kidder

Issue/ Problem	Dilemma	Distress	Temptation	Silence
Important values present	Two alternative courses of action: Right vs. Right decision	The right course of action is known but the clinician cannot perform it	Choice between right and wrong	Values are challenged but no one is speaking about this challenge to values

The Situation: _____

Rationale:

Ethical Principles and/or Standards of Ethical Conduct of the PTA (see Appendixes A and B)

Code of Ethics (Principles) for PTs	Rationale	Standards of Ethical Conduct (Standards) for PTAs	Rationale

Suggested Action:

Case Example 4

ALL THAT IS NEW AND SHINY
Conflict of Intertest- Benefit

Physical therapists embrace cutting edge changes in health care, seeking to use our unique observation skills and movement analysis ability to offer patients the best in individual, appropriate safe and effective treatment. PTs are always seeking ways in which to enhance and improve access to care. Technology provides many opportunities for cutting edge treatment, at the same time it raises ethical questions that should be considered when determining the best plan of care for a patient.

Paul and Lindsey pride themselves on a practice that provides quality care to all of their patients and is well respected in the community. They vowed when they started working together that they would challenge each other and constantly strive to maintain a quality state of the art practice. Consistent with their vision statement, their practice is always prepared to provide their patients with "practice innovation." Both Paul and Lindsey have their OCS and continue to analyze their practice to determine what they should offer to best meet the needs of their patients. In 2020 they transitioned rapidly to telehealth to provide access to the services required by their patients, and when they returned to in person care there were elements of telehealth that they maintained realizing how beneficial it was for their patients to have access to physical therapy on terms that best met their needs. Paul and Lindsey were well known in the PT community through their work with the local University DPT program. They have published their work on the treatment of a variety of musculoskeletal conditions and are well regarded for their outcomes.

It wasn't much of a surprise when they were contacted by a company that was expanding into the area of digital physical therapy and they were seeking to gauge the interest of Paul and Lindsey in becoming part of their team of therapists. Neither knew too much about digital PT other than the little they had read in the media about this fast-growing trending practice. They were aware that the digital companies were partnering with large insurers to offer what they called "simple physical therapy" for musculoskeletal conditions. Paul and Lindsey had been looking for ways in which to expand their practice footprint and were open to various alternatives. They had to admit that they were curious enough to want to know more, so they agreed to meet with a representative of the company. The following week they met with the CEO Seth virtually and he gave them a good idea of the PT services they were implementing. He was quick to point out that it is a physical therapist who meets with the patient, and quickly allayed their fears by ensuring that their company only allowed PTs to interact with patients. They were all aware that some of the companies springing up in the digital space utilized health coaches or health monitors who were not physical therapists, yet they were very liberal in using the terminology physical therapy which is a protected term in most jurisdictions. Having crossed that question off of their long list of queries, they were curious about the technology and how the software was used. Seth explained that the therapist conducted a digital assessment and then the PT created a customized treatment plan. Each patient uses an app which monitors what the patient is doing and also provides them with exercises that the PT selected. The exercises have clear 3D animation and voice narration to help the patient do them correctly. They also get paper copies of exercises to provide guidance. Seth concluded his description of the plan of care pointing out that follow up with the patient is either through video visits or live chats and the app provides ongoing information regarding the patient's level of participation in the program. Paul and Lindsey were impressed with how the technology was used but they had questions that they posed to Seth, hoping to get a better sense of whether the standard of care they prided themselves on maintaining could continue to be met. Seth was anxious to hear their questions. They began with a concern about professional responsibility. If they felt a patient could not safely be treated with a completely remote program what was available for them to refer and hand off the patient to a qualified physical therapist in the patient's local area? Seth's response was that, of course they should not treat a patient that they do not believe is a good candidate for physical therapy interventions. Their next question was somewhat related, what if the patient was not an appropriate referral? The patient did not need the skilled services of a physical therapist, was there any expectation that they continue to provide care, because the insurance company had purchased the service and made it available to all of their insured … was there a contract driven obligation to treat? Seth was not quite sure what the answer was but did encourage them to "broaden their outlook" since doesn't everyone need physical therapy? Paul and Lindsey could not argue that a lot of people do need physical therapy that do not get it, however the skilled services of a PT may not be needed by everyone *all* the time. It is the professional discretion of the PT to determine the appropriateness of care. Paul and Lindsey were licensed in their home state, and each carried one additional license linked to the state where they went to school that they had on inactive status, but it was easy enough to reactivate. but how were they to manage the potential of patients located in the other states where they did not hold a license? Seth was impressed, many of the people he had been speaking with about this opportunity did not even consider state licensure. Seth assured them that the company did try to match clients with licensed clinicians, and the company would encourage them, if they want to drive up their referral volume to take advantage of the fact that their state was a part of the licensure contract. He suggested that they should apply to get privileges in as many states as they possibly could. However, Seth said they would try to only send referrals for individuals in the states where they are licensed but ultimately the decision to accept the case was theirs. Paul and Lindsey were pretty sure they had a lot more questions to ask …. but certainly they had a lot to think about with the information at hand.

CONSIDER AND REFLECT

When faced with changes in practice every physical therapist has to consider the scope of practice from three aspects. Is what they are planning to engage in part of the professional scope of physical therapy? Is it within the regulatory scope in their jurisdiction and are they sufficiently proficient in the intervention to determine that it is within their individual scope of practice. Is what they are doing cost effective and beneficial to the patient? In short are they willingly accepting responsibility for their actions, the essence of accountability.

After working through the ethical decision-making process, what course of action would you suggest?

Ethical Decision-Making Worksheet

Case: _____

The Realm   Jack Glaser (1994)

Individual	Organizational/ Institutional	Societal
The good of the patient/ client and focuses on rights, duties, relationships and behaviors between individuals	Good of the organization, focuses on structures and systems, which facilitate organizational or institutional goals	Concerned with the common good

(continued on following page)

The Realm _____

Rationale:

The Individual Process: James Rest (1994, 1999)

Moral Sensitivity	Moral Judgment	Moral Motivation	Moral Courage	Moral Potency (Hannah and Avolio, 2010)
Recognizing, interpreting, and framing an ethical situation	Right versus wrong actions. Generating options, selecting and applying ethical principles	Priority on ethical values over other values. Professionalism is a primary motivator for ethical behavior	Implementing the chosen ethical action, development of a plan	Includes decision making that includes moral ownership, courage, and self-efficacy

The Individual Process: _____

Rationale:

The Situation   Swisher et al. (2005) adapted from Kidder

Issue/ Problem	Dilemma	Distress	Temptation	Silence
Important values present	Two alternative courses of action: Right vs. Right decision	The right course of action is known but the clinician cannot perform it	Choice between right and wrong	Values are challenged but no one is speaking about this challenge to values

The Situation: _____

Rationale: _____

_____

_____

Ethical Principles and/or Standards of Ethical Conduct of the PTA (see Appendixes A and B)

Code of Ethics (Principles) for PTs	Rationale	Standards of Ethical Conduct (Standards) for PTAs	Rationale

Suggested Action:

CHAPTER 12

Boundary Issues

It is the very nature of physical therapy to become very close with patients. As a health-care professional, we are granted a license to touch other people. There is a delicate balance between the important interpersonal relationship developed between the therapist and their patient while still maintaining the necessary boundary that reinforces the integrity of the patient–therapist relationship. At the core of this relationship is trust and that is another reason why the boundary must be defined. There are many potential opportunities for boundary crossings. Some of them are just a small crossing of the line such as accepting an invitation to an event hosted by a patient, and returning to the "safe side" of the line is easy to do. Other boundary crossings are quite egregious and obviously inappropriate such as having intimate relationships with a patient. There is a definite professional barrier to returning to the appropriate side of the line. Another common boundary issue in PT is managing **dual relationships**, the patient who is also the therapist's friend. The patient's family member or the patient who the PT or PTA becomes romantically involved with. The ultimate responsibility for maintaining a professional relationship belongs with the therapist. It is not always the therapist who crosses boundaries. Sometimes, it is the patient who crosses the line; however, the responsibility to maintain professional limits still is the responsibility of the therapist. Confounding boundary issues is also the responsibility of the therapist to recognize the potential for a power gradient issue. The physical therapist by virtue of their role has power and must have the self-awareness to recognize when that power could be used inappropriately or misinterpreted by a patient.

A Family Affair	**A dual relationship**
Who Sent *Me* a Text?	**Social media boundary violation**
Movement Specialist Redefined	**Power gradient**
With all best intentions	**Informed consent**

Case Example 5

A FAMILY AFFAIR
A dual relationship

It's the goal of every PT to ensure that his or her patients receive the best possible care. But what if a prospective patient is the PT's spouse, and the PT is the best option among local PTs for his spouse's particular physical condition? Consider the following scenario.

Larry has focused his entire career as a PT on issues related to the cervical spine, as he has long been fascinated by the mechanical challenges of its role supporting the head. Accordingly, Larry is a board-certified orthopedic clinical specialist. In addition to serving this patient population in his solo private practice, he is a credentialed clinical instructor who offers at least two rotations a year to Doctor of Physical Therapy students interested in taking a very manual approach to patient care.

Larry is also quite active in the community as a youth soccer coach, Boy Scout leader, Special Olympics volunteer, and accessibility consultant to the town planning board. In short, he's quite well known and respected in the community, and his practice is thriving. This is mostly good, except in a few cases in which people have infringed on the lines separating Larry's professional relationship with the individual from his personal one. Occasionally, a parent who Larry knows through youth soccer has become his patient and has come by Larry's house in the evening to ask him to review aspects of his or her home-exercise program. A few times, his neighbors have sought Larry out on a weekend for a gratis "consultation" about their latest ache or pain. While Larry is always friendly, he typically asks such visitors to schedule an appointment and stop by his office if they need more than a simple clarification or a quick piece of advice.

One winter day, Larry's wife, Cheryl, is involved in a fender-bender on an icy road. At first, she seems to be uninjured, but within 48 hours she is experiencing cervical pain, with an accompanying headache. Over-the-counter analgesics and ice aren't helping her, and Larry notes postural changes that are consistent with soft-tissue injury. At his urging, Cheryl gets complete workup from the couple's primary care physician to rule out any other pathology. She is then cleared to begin physical therapy.

The question for Larry now is whether he should be the PT to treat Cheryl. On the one hand, issues of the cervical spine are his specialty, and he's certain that he is the best PT in the area to treat her particular condition. (Typically, after all, other PTs in the community refer their patients to him who have cervical problems.) On the other hand, however, this is his wife who Larry is considering taking on as a patient.

There's a clause in the couple's insurance policy advising him against taking on family members as patients without well-documented justification for the decision. While Larry is certain that he can justify the treatment of Cheryl to the company's satisfaction, he understands the reasoning. The insurance company is wary that familial relationships may lead to unnecessary and costlier care, due to the provider's abundance of care and caution for a loved one. Can he be completely objective in his treatment of Cheryl? Larry believes that he can, but still to do something about taking on his wife as his patient doesn't feel quite right to him.

Sitting in his living room, he hears his wife groan in the kitchen, and knows that she needs the services of a physical therapist sooner rather than later. There are several excellent PTs in the community, albeit none who are as skilled as he in issues of the cervical spine. Should Larry entrust Cheryl's care to one of those other PTs, or treat her himself? He knows he must decide tonight.

CONSIDER AND REFLECT

Larry wishes his decision was black and white. If he and Cheryl lived in a rural area that was not served by other PTs, then he wouldn't hesitate to treat her himself. Conversely, if he had a practice partner whose own background and experience matched his own in treating issues of the cervical spine, he most certainly would refer Cheryl's care to that individual. As it is, he firmly believes that he is the best PT to treat his wife's condition, but he's hesitant to do so.

If Larry reviews his ethical obligations as a PT, he'll find that, while there is no specific principle regarding treatment of family members, a number of principles have bearing on his situation and can collectively lead him to the optimal decision.

Larry believes that the optimal outcome in this situation is for Cheryl to be treated by a PT whose knowledge and skills treating cervical spine issues match his own. That outcome is not available, however, leaving Larry to determine the next-best possible course of action given the ethical considerations involved.

After working through the ethical decision-making process, what course of action would you suggest?

Ethical Decision-Making Worksheet

Case: _____

The Realm

Jack Glaser (1994)

Individual	Organizational/ Institutional	Societal
The good of the patient/ client and focuses on rights, duties, relationships, and behaviors between individuals	Good of the organization, focuses on structures and systems, which facilitate organizational or institutional goals	Concerned with the common good

The Realm: _____

Rationale:

(continued on following page)

The Individual Process   James Rest (1994, 1999)

Moral Sensitivity	Moral Judgment	Moral Motivation	Moral Courage	Moral Potency (Hannah and Avolio, 2010)
Recognizing, interpreting, and framing an ethical situation	Right vs. wrong actions. Generating options, selecting and applying ethical principles	Priority on ethical values over other values. Professionalism is a primary motivator for ethical behavior	Implementing the chosen ethical action, development of a plan	Includes decision making that includes moral ownership, courage, and self-efficacy

The Individual Process: _____

Rationale:

The Situation: Swisher et al. (2005) adapted from Kidder

Issue/ Problem	Dilemma	Distress	Temptation	Silence
Important values present	Two alternative courses of action: Right vs. Right decision	The right course of action is known but the clinician cannot perform it	Choice between right and wrong	Values are challenged but no one is speaking about this challenge to values

The Situation: _____

Rationale:

Ethical Principles and/or Standards of Ethical Conduct of the PTA (see Appendixes A and B)

Code of Ethics (Principles) for PTs	Rationale	Standards of Ethical Conduct (Standards) for PTAs	Rationale

(continued on following page)

Code of Ethics (Principles) for PTs	Rationale	Standards of Ethical Conduct (Standards) for PTAs	Rationale

Suggested Action:

Case Example 6

WHO SENT *ME* A TEXT?
The conundrum of social media

F-r-i-e-n-d. Six letters that can mean a lot—or not so much. Consider the following scenario, in which a simple request is weighted with potential ramifications.

As the youngest and newest PT at his clinic, Jeff is used to being the "go-to-guy" for some of the older and less tech-savvy PTs on staff when it comes to issues related to Internet technology (IT) and social media. He has helped several PTs shape their personal Facebook pages, led a staff in-service on Twitter, and contributes to the private practice's website, in-house blog, Facebook page, and Twitter feed.

Jeff tries to keep his personal presence on social media separate from his professional one. While on his personal page he is "Facebook friends" with some of his coworkers and even with a few former patients (with a caveat that will be discussed shortly), he makes it a rule never to discuss anything work-related in those interactions. He keeps up with the lives of selected work friends just as he would with any other friend on Facebook. Jeff's personal policy is to turn down friend requests from former or current patients—thanking them for their interest but politely explaining that he would prefer to keep the relationship strictly professional. (He knows, too, that former patients may well become future ones.)

There are a few exceptions that come with asterisks—former patients with whom Jeff has become both Facebook and full-fledged friends through shared interests in skiing and/or golf, Jeff's biggest recreational passions. A couple of his former patients are, like Jeff, members of the local ski club. Two other former patients are members of the golf club to which Jeff belongs. A fifth former patient belongs to both groups; Jeff now considers him to be a close friend.

One day, Jeff receives via Facebook a friend request from a recent patient named Michael, who had presented with several comorbidities and made great progress while he was under Jeff's care. Michael sometimes made Jeff uncomfortable, however, by, in Jeff's view, over sharing about his personal life. During one visit he told Jeff that he often feels insecure and defensive, that he has few friends, and that he gets depressed when he feels that his overtures of friendship have been rebuffed. On another occasion he told Jeff that he's "been told" he can be pushy and needy, but that he finds it difficult to back off.

Jeff does not know whether Michael ever has seen a mental health professional, but he suspects the possibility from some allusions Michael has made. Jeff never encouraged or sought to prolong these personal lines of conversation when Michael introduced them. He typically tried, rather, to refocus Jeff on his physical therapy and the movement issues on which Michael and he were working.

On this final visit for physical therapy, Michael pointed to a photo on Jeff's desk of the PT standing on a golf course with his clubs and remarked out of the blue "I really like you. You should teach me to play sometime."

Jeff had responded lightly, "Golf will break your heart! Get out before you even start my friend. That's my advice to you."

Jeff replays that conversation as he views the Facebook friend request on his computer screen. Could Michael have imbued Jeff's innocuous word choice with unintended meaning?

In this particular case, Jeff is reluctant to proceed as he typically does—explaining his reasoning and declining Michael's Facebook request. He doesn't really know *what* to do. So, at first, he does nothing. He hopes the request has no outsized meaning for Michael. Maybe it's just one of many "friend" requests Michael has made, and Michael won't pursue it further.

The next day, however, Jeff returns to his office after lunch to find a voicemail message from Michael asking if he'd received the email from Facebook. The PT realizes at that moment that he's probably going to have to engage Michael on the subject. But he isn't sure what exactly to say or write to Michael—recalling how deeply affected his former patient had seemed to be by the perceived rejections he'd recounted during his physical therapy visits. Jeff doesn't immediately respond to the phone message, either, unrealistically hoping—but hoping nonetheless—that Michael's inquiries will end there.

Unsurprisingly, however, when Jeff checks his email between patient visits the following morning, he finds that he's received a message; he finds that he's received a message from Michael that reads, simply, "Left you a phone message. Please check." There's also an automated message from

Facebook reminding Jeff that Michael had sent him a friend request the day before.

Jeff slumps down in his office chair. He doesn't want to further dent Michael's self-esteem, but neither does he wish to engage in this way with a former patient. He also worries about leading Michael on, in a sense, as he has reason to believe that his former patient may equate Facebook friendship with a real, multidimensional relationship. How to let him down gently?

Or, should he let him down at all? Could a Facebook friendship with Michael "work"? Might his professional/personal rule of thumb toward social media, Jeff wonders, be a little too rigid?

His phone buzzes, alerting him that his next patient has arrived. As he exits his office, he eyes copies of Physical Therapy on his bookshelf, which reminds him that he can draw on APTA resources in considering his course of action. He resolves to explore the association's website at lunchtime to see what guidance the Code of Ethics for the Physical Therapist might offer him, and whether any other APTA documents shed additional light.

CONSIDER AND REFLECT

Jeff must determine whether to respond to Michael's Facebook friend request in the same manner as he has addressed past requests from other former patients, or whether to accept the request as, essentially, a goodwill gesture to a patient who Jeff believes has emotional issues.

Jeff will find the APTA's Code of Ethics for the Physical Therapist useful, as well as the APTA document Standards of Conduct in the Use of Social Media. He and his colleagues may also consider using those documents as blueprints for crafting a practice-wide policy on the use of social media in all its facets.

Ethical Decision-Making Worksheet

Case: _____

The Realm   Jack Glaser (1994)

Individual	Organizational/ Institutional	Societal
The good of the patient/client and focuses on rights, duties, relationships, and behaviors between individuals	Good of the organization, focuses on structures and systems, which facilitate organizational or institutional goals	Concerned with the common good

(continued on following page)

The Realm: _____

Rationale:

The Individual Process   James Rest (1994, 1999)

Moral Sensitivity	Moral Judgment	Moral Motivation	Moral Courage	Moral Potency (Hannah and Avolio, 2010)
Recognizing, interpreting, and framing an ethical situation	Right vs. wrong actions. Generating options, selecting and applying ethical principles	Priority on ethical values over other values. Professionalism is a primary motivator for ethical behavior	Implementing the chosen ethical action, development of a plan	Includes decision making that includes moral ownership, courage, and self-efficacy

The Individual Process: _____

Rationale:

The Situation: Swisher et al. (2005) adapted from Kidder

Issue/ Problem	Dilemma	Distress	Temptation	Silence
Important values present	Two alternative courses of action: Right vs. Right decision	The right course of action is known but the clinician cannot perform it	Choice between right and wrong	Values are challenged but no one is speaking about this challenge to values

The Situation: _____

Rationale:

Ethical Principles and/or Standards of Ethical Conduct of the PTA (see Appendixes A and B)

Code of Ethics (Principles) for PTs	Rationale	Standards of Ethical Conduct (Standards) for PTAs	Rationale

(continued on following page)

Code of Ethics (Principles) for PTs	Rationale	Standards of Ethical Conduct (Standards) for PTAs	Rationale

Suggested Action:

Case Example 7

MOVEMENT SPECIALIST REDEFINED
Power gradient

One of the most important professional activities that a physical therapist or physical therapist assistant can be involved with is the clinical education of future colleagues. The cross between mentor, educator, friend, critic, and role model describes how the student sees the clinical instructor. With all these roles, the clinician needs to recognize their duty to the student and the importance of maintaining a professional relationship.

Jim makes a point to sign up for at least one student physical therapist a year. While it takes a lot of time, he feels strongly that it is a professional responsibility. He gratefully remembers his clinical instructors while he was in school and wants to "pay it forward" providing a quality experience for a student. The other therapists in the large rehabilitation hospital where he works also consider the student program a significant way in which to be engaged with the profession. Tom, his new third-year student from State, is starting his final clinical rotation. Jim and Tom hit it off immediately and Jim begins to orient Tom to the patients and the routine at the hospital, generally a rather steep learning curve in this very busy clinical environment where every patient is complex. It is not unusual for students assigned to this facility to have difficulty; it is known to be quite challenging. While the days are busy, the two men find a few minutes to discuss the sports headlines and banter about the prospects for the upcoming season. Unfortunately, Jim finds that Tom is not prepared for the neurological case load that Jim is treating. Jim is willing to help Tom and both men come in early and stay late, but Tom is still struggling. He is in contact with the school, and the Director of Clinical Education visited the facility to work with Tom and Jim. They determine that a learning contract should be put in place, so it is very clear to all what is expected of Tom to successfully complete this clinical rotation. Though he was having difficulty and Jim still was unable to give him the caseload he should be carrying, they still had a very good working relationship. During lunch break on Friday Jim shares with Tom that he and his wife are moving from their apartment to their new house and one of his friends that was going to help with the move was sick. Jim suddenly looks at Tom and without seemingly stopping to think he says to Tom, "hey I've taught you everything you need to know about body mechanics, can you give me a hand?" Tom did have weekend plans, but he is pretty sure that everybody will understand the importance of helping out his CI. He sees it as an opportunity to help his CI who has been so good to him … yet he is concerned that it could appear that he just trying to "butter up" his CI. He didn't see he had much choice … so Tom willingly agrees to help out, spending both Saturday and Sunday as Jim's "right hand man." Monday morning Tom and two of the other students who were at the clinical site compared their weekend activities. When Tom shares with them that he helped Jim all weekend they exchange a knowing glance, passing the comment "that should ensure a passing grade" before going off to start their day.

CONSIDER AND REFLECT

Jim the CI appears to be unaware of the boundary crossing that he creates when he asks his student Tom to assist him, he is also unaware that he had power over Tom and gave little choice but to willingly assist him. The fact that Tom is struggling complicates the situation, is there any potential for favoritism? Even the appearance of favoritism can have very negative consequences.

After working through the ethical decision-making process, what course of action would you suggest?

Ethical Decision-Making Worksheet

Case: _____

The Realm   Jack Glaser (1994)

Individual	Organizational/Institutional	Societal
The good of the patient/client and focuses on rights, duties, relationships, and behaviors between individuals	Good of the organization, focuses on structures and systems, which facilitate organizational or institutional goals	Concerned with the common good

(continued on following page)

The Realm: _____

Rationale:

The Individual Process

James Rest (1994, 1999)

Moral Sensitivity	Moral Judgment	Moral Motivation	Moral Courage	Moral Potency (Hannah and Avolio, 2010)
Recognizing, interpreting, and framing an ethical situation	Right vs. wrong actions. Generating options, selecting and applying ethical principles	Priority on ethical values over other values. Professionalism is a primary motivator for ethical behavior	Implementing the chosen ethical action, development of a plan	Includes decision making that includes moral ownership, courage, and self-efficacy

The Individual Process: _____

Rationale:

The Situation

Swisher et al. (2005) adapted from Kidder

Issue/ Problem	Dilemma	Distress	Temptation	Silence
Important values present	Two alternative courses of action: Right vs. Right decision	The right course of action is known but the clinician cannot perform it	Choice between right and wrong	Values are challenged but no one is speaking about this challenge to values

The Situation: _____

Rationale:

Ethical Principles and/or Standards of Ethical Conduct of the PTA (see Appendixes A and B)

Code of Ethics (Principles) for PTs	Rationale	Standards of Ethical Conduct (Standards) for PTAs	Rationale

(continued on following page)

Code of Ethics (Principles) for PTs	Rationale	Standards of Ethical Conduct (Standards) for PTAs	Rationale

Suggested Action:

Case Example 8

WITH ALL BEST INTENTIONS:
When consent is not informed.

Rich has always been a physical therapist who was a dedicated "Lifelong Learner." He is passionate about keeping up with the growth of the profession and always aware of any new intervention or treatment strategy that he can explore the information about and determine its efficacy in patient care. His bottom line is always striving to determine what will benefit will benefit a patient. He attends as many continuing education courses that he can, and reads multiple journals across disciplines to improve and expand his clinical skills. He is more than willing to share his knowledge and expertise with colleagues and his favorite time is "anytime" he can delve into a patient problem and pull out something from his continuously growing index of care that will benefit his patient or those of his colleagues. Rich has a new patient, Lorraine, who fell on her coccyx and has been experiencing significant pain for weeks. She did attend physical therapy and had some minimal relief but was not progressing and still in considerable pain, so she made an appointment with Rich because she heard about his excellent patient outcomes on social media. In contemplating seeing this patient he considered the article that he read about a technique which involves internally manipulating the coccyx to reposition it into its normal position, he does further research, looking in depth at the hands-on skills he needs to successfully execute the manipulation. He feels confident that he will be able to do it. The patient is a good historian, providing an accurate medical history and a good description of the mechanism of injury. He decides that his patient is a perfect candidate for this intervention. He says to the patient he would like to try "something new" with her. The patient says she is willing to try anything he suggests after all that is why she came to him. Rich casually asks her if she would like to have a chaperone in the room during the procedure. The patient seems a bit startled by that and does not answer right away. Rich takes her silence to mean, it is OK to continue and with that, Rich proceeds to provide the intervention. The patient does not object, but she does become very quiet. Rich is concentrating intensely, making sure that he executes the procedure exactly as he saw it demonstrated so he does not harm the patient. After the session, when Rich asks the patient how she is feeling, she shares that the pain has decreased and leaves without making another appointment, she tells the receptionist "She will call." Rich was very excited that he was able to help this patient, so he is extremely surprised the next day when law enforcement shows up at his office to arrest him for sexual assault as reported by his patient, Lorraine.

CONSIDER AND REFLECT

Rich is anxious to help not just Lorraine but every patient he has the privilege to treat. He is passionate about his ability to impact patients in a positive way. While his intentions are admirable, he missed some very important messages that his patient was sending him, and he did not provide the patient with true informed consent. Think of things that he could have done to help his patient understand and benefit from the care he was so anxious to be able to provide.

After working through the ethical decision-making process, what course of action would you suggest?

Ethical Decision-Making Worksheet

Case: _____

The Realm   Jack Glaser (1994)

Individual	Organizational/ Institutional	Societal
The good of the patient/client and focuses on rights, duties, relationships, and behaviors between individuals	Good of the organization, focuses on structures and systems, which facilitate organizational or institutional goals	Concerned with the common good

(continued on following page)

The Realm: _____

Rationale:

The Individual Process   James Rest (1994, 1999)

Moral Sensitivity	Moral Judgment	Moral Motivation	Moral Courage	Moral Potency (Hannah and Avolio, 2010)
Recognizing, interpreting, and framing an ethical situation	Right vs. wrong actions. Generating options, selecting and applying ethical principles	Priority on ethical values over other values. Professionalism is a primary motivator for ethical behavior	Implementing the chosen ethical action, development of a plan	Includes decision making that includes moral ownership, courage, and self-efficacy

The Individual Process: _____

Rationale:

The Situation   Swisher et al. (2005) adapted from Kidder

Issue/ Problem	Dilemma	Distress	Temptation	Silence
Important values present	Two alternative courses of action: Right vs. Right decision	The right course of action is known but the clinician cannot perform it	Choice between right and wrong	Values are challenged but no one is speaking about this challenge to values

The Situation: _____

Rationale:

Ethical Principles and/or Standards of Ethical Conduct of the PTA (see Appendixes A and B)

Code of Ethics (Principles) for PTs	Rationale	Standards of Ethical Conduct (Standards) for PTAs	Rationale

(continued on following page)

Code of Ethics (Principles) for PTs	Rationale	Standards of Ethical Conduct (Standards) for PTAs	Rationale

Suggested Action:

CHAPTER 13

Practice Issues

Physical therapists (PTs) have a broad scope of practice treating across all organ systems, and patients are seen by physical therapists across the entire lifespan. Physical therapist assistants (PTAs) have an equally broad scope of work. In addition, the venues in which physical therapy is delivered are only limited by the imagination. PTs and PTAs practice in traditional settings such as hospitals and private practices and less traditional settings such as industry, sports, and the space program. Regardless of setting the responsibilities of the physical therapist are guided by the standards of the profession such as the Code of Ethics and the Guide to Ethical Conduct. Practice settings are not necessarily subject to professional standards, but PTs and PTAs that practice in those settings are most definitely subject to professional guidance and this guidance goes across all practice settings. The PT and the PTA ultimately hold the license and have the professional responsibility to uphold the integrity of that license. They may find themselves working in an environment that challenges their professional values and integrity. They ultimately have to determine if they can work in that environment and maintain their integrity, or they must seek to effect change to make it possible to remain or they must consider the professional guidance in Principle 7 that cautions against remaining in a setting that prevents a physical therapist from fulfilling professional obligations to patients/clients.

Can You "See" Me Now?	**Workplace dictating a service delivery model**
Put Me In, Coach	**The complexities of answering to patient and employer expectations simultaneously**
Are You the PT for Me?	**Self-assessment to determine what is best for the patient**

Case Example 9

CAN YOU "SEE" ME NOW?
Workplace dictating a service delivery model

Advances in technology are changing the face of healthcare, but there are limits to what it can achieve—particularly if it is applied inappropriately. Consider this scenario, in which a physical therapist (PT) is asked to do something he strongly feels is ethically and clinically wrong.

Sam has been a PT for more than thirty years, practicing in a variety of settings. Two months ago, when he moved from the East Coast to live closer to his aging mother and father, he signed on at a private practice named Active Corps. There, he has enjoyed the patients, his work, and his colleagues—with one exception. His supervisor, Becky, who is not a PT, often gives him a hard time for what she calls his "old-school" ways, and sometimes questions whether he's a "team player."

As Sam sees it, "old-school" means "slow" and sometimes "less-profitable" to Becky, whereas it means "cautious," "deliberate," and "patient-centered" to him. He thinks of himself as a team player—with the patient at quarterback, as the reason that the team exists. In most contexts, Sam takes pride in being called old-school. But Becky clearly doesn't mean it as a compliment.

Sam and Becky have had their arguments, but to date she has grudgingly supported all of his practice rationales and treatment decisions. Veteran PTs on staff assure him that Becky is "all bark and no bite" and tell him that they, too, have had disagreements with her that have been resolved without patient care being compromised in any way.

One day, however, Becky hands Sam a patient file and says, "Scott Jones was a patient of ours, on and off, until he moved to Arizona a couple of years ago. He's a funny guy. He called me around this time last year just to say, 'I think the move has done my body wonders, because I haven't seen a PT in 18 months! I miss you guys, but I don't miss the treatment and the exercise!' But then, just the other day, he called again and said, 'Beck, I guess nothing lasts forever. I've had a flare-up of cervical pain and had to restart my old home program. But I'm not sure I'm doing it right, so I'm going to need some help. I could go to a PT here, but I'd rather stick with the folks I know and trust.'"

"Okay," Sam says. "So, you want me to see Mr Jones?"

"Exactly," Becky replies.

"Great," Sam responds. "When's he going to be in town?" (Scott Jones's new home is about a 6-hour drive away.) "I'll check my schedule and see when we can slide him in."

"That's the beauty of it," Becky says. "He won't be in town at all, but he'd still rather give us his business than someone there in Arizona. I figure you can just Skype with him. After all, you've got his patient record, and he can show you how he's been doing his exercises. Set him straight, and that'll be it. Quick and easy! He makes the adjustments and we retain a happy customer and bill him for a telehealth visit. Talk about a win-win!"

Sam is taken aback. His first thought is that nobody "wins" when he's unable to evaluate a patient appropriately to determine whether his old home program addresses the current "flare-up." Never mind the fact that Active Corps has not engaged in telehealth before, and Sam isn't familiar with what, if anything, his state practice act says about PTs' eligibility to use telehealth in practice.

"I really think we'll need to have Mr Jones come here for a look," Sam says. "Either that, or he should see a PT close to home who can properly evaluate precisely what's going on and what needs to be done about it."

Becky looks impatient. "I think I know what this is all about," she says. "You went to school in a different day. But trust me, the technology's easy. My son is in the Marines, and I Skype with him all the time. I'll show you how to do it. Don't worry about it."

Sam inwardly seethes now, as Becky had just added ageist insult to a plan that could cause patient injury. Just last week, in fact, Sam had discussed with a couple of his Active Corps colleagues a journal article about technology and techniques being used in distance evaluation by physiotherapists in Australia and New Zealand. Sam recalls how a colleague had remarked, "That's a great example of the kind of reach PTs can have when they have the right technology and training."

Sam tries to calm his nerves and choose his words carefully. "What you're talking about would be great," he says in a measured tone, "but it's a little more complicated than a simple home-exercise tune-up. While it's true that some impressive things are being done these days in distance evaluation, I don't believe—"

Becky cuts him off, and Sam can tell she's getting angry. "I'm not talking about doing an *evaluation*," she sputters. "Were you not listening to me? Scott Jones has had this problem before! All you need to do is ask him to demonstrate what he's been doing, look at the notes in his file, and tell him if he's on target. No muss, no fuss."

What she's saying is wrong on so many levels that Sam hardly knows how to respond. Finally, he latches onto an aspect of his dilemma that she perhaps will appreciate.

"Becky," he says, "I'm not licensed in the state of Arizona."

"What does *licensing* have to do with it?" she angrily retorts. "You're licensed *here*! And you're just talking to him on the *phone*!"

Words fail Sam at that point. He finds himself simply shaking his head "No."

"I'm sorry you feel this way," his supervisor says, "but if you're unwilling to treat a patient you've been assigned, I may have to replace you with a PT who will. Need I remind you that it's a buyer's job market?"

CONSIDER AND REFLECT

Far from being the recalcitrant Luddite Becky paints him as being, Sam is excited about technology's promise for physical therapy. But it must be used appropriately, in ways that are prudent, legal, and best serve the patient. What Becky is demanding he does meets none of those criteria. Becky is suggesting that the patient does not need an initial evaluation. Why is she suggesting that this patient get substandard care? Sam feels that he can't possibly comply. The area is flooded with PTs, however, and he needs a local job to be able to tend to his mother and father's needs. What do you think Sam should do?

After working through the ethical decision-making process, what course of action would you suggest?

Ethical Decision-Making Worksheet

Case: _____

The Realm   Jack Glaser (1994)

Individual	Organizational/ Institutional	Societal
The good of the patient/ client and focuses on rights, duties, relationships, and behaviors between individuals	Good of the organization, focuses on structures and systems, which facilitate organizational or institutional goals	Concern with the common good

The Realm: _____

Rationale:

The Individual Process   James Rest (1994, 1999)

Moral Sensitivity	Moral Judgment	Moral Motivation	Moral Courage	Moral Potency (Hannah and Avolio, 2010)
Recognizing, interpreting, and framing an ethical situation	Right vs. wrong actions. Generating options, selecting and applying ethical principles	Priority on ethical values over other values. Professionalism is a primary motivator for ethical behavior	Implementing the chosen ethical action, development of a plan	Includes decision making that includes moral ownership, courage, and self-efficacy

(continued on following page)

The Individual Process:_____

Rationale:

The Situation   Swisher et al. (2005) adapted from Kidder

Issue/ Problem	Dilemma	Distress	Temptation	Silence
Important values present	Two alternative courses of action: Right vs. Right decision	The right course of action is known but the clinician cannot perform it	Choice between right and wrong	Values are challenged but no one is speaking about this challenge to values

The Situation: _____

Rationale: .

Ethical Principles and/or Standards of Ethical Conduct of the PTA (see Appendixes A and B)

Code of Ethics (Principles) for PTs	Rationale	Standards of Ethical Conduct (Standards) for PTAs	Rationale

Suggested Action:

Case Example 10

PUT ME IN, COACH
The complexities of answering patient and employer expectations simultaneously

Physical therapists are responsible for making appropriate decisions in the patient's best interest at all times, but there are times when the patient's best interest and the interests of other closely associated interested parties may conflict. The recent discussions regarding sports injuries and the ability to return to play safely have sparked much interest in the ethical conflicts that may arise when making decisions "in the best interest."

John is a physical therapist who works for a professional football team in the National Football League. He has a signed contract with the team to provide rehabilitation services. The position with the NFL team provides him with valuable prestige to market his services in his own private practice. He works closely with the team physician an orthopedic surgeon to rehabilitate athletes to return to play. He has a good relationship with the team coaches particularly the head coach who trusts his judgment in returning players safely but as quickly as possible to play.

Recently, Nick the team's star running back was referred to John to strengthen the lower extremity muscles after Nick underwent a partial meniscectomy in his right knee. The surgery was performed twelve days ago. John's goal is to strengthen the muscles in the right lower leg, particularly the quadriceps muscle. Evidence-based guidelines indicate that quadriceps isokinetic concentric peak torque and power output should be within 90% of the contralateral leg; with a 60% hamstring to quadriceps power ratio in the involved leg (Zviliac et al., 2014). John is well aware that to return to sport, particularly one with high demands, without these strength parameters may be unsafe and detrimental to the long-term health of the athlete. John takes the responsibility of monitoring the players' fitness to play very seriously.

Although the head coach trusts John's judgment, he has been particularly eager to return this athlete to play because of the playoff game upcoming in one week. The athlete himself wants to return as soon as possible but expressed to John on more than one occasion that he wants to make sure that he is completely healthy and ready before returning to play. Based on the standard evidence-based protocol, John started slowly, systematically progressing Nick's strengthening regime while controlling for pain and swelling and some loss of motion. Though John picked up the pace very early in the program, it did not seem fast enough for his colleagues. Much to the dismay of the head coach, team owner, and team physician, based on his ongoing evaluations John has not yet progressed Nick to low and high velocity concentric isokinetic training. On more than one occasion during the day, the head coach catches up with John in the training room questioning why Nick's progress is so slow and reminding John that the big game is only five days away. In fact, the head coach and team physician observing rehabilitation, both asked Nick why he wasn't being more aggressive in his strength training, telling him "Nick we and your teammates are counting on you to be ready to play next Sunday." John overhears this and isn't surprised when Nick asks him if he can "speed up the process a bit, explaining the team is on my case." He does remind John that he continues to experience some pain and swelling in his knee. John is well aware that he has already been pushing Nick, probably harder than is dictated by his best professional judgment adding another treatment session to those he is already participating in and starting the low and high velocity strength training that normally he would delay just a little longer. He is confident, but Nick is tolerating the changes and assures himself that it is to be expected that he would have some pain.

Nick tells John, "I trust your judgment so I will try to work through the pain and swelling during these exercises. I know you wouldn't suggest anything that is not in my best interest." John feels guilty about pushing Nick so hard, but he is also sensitive to the pressure from team management and coaches. If he can just get Nick ready, it will benefit the entire team. Nick has made excellent progress. As he is one tough guy, there is no wonder why he is so successful on the field. In spite of his positive thoughts, John can't help but think in whose best interest are his clinical judgments made?

CONSIDER AND REFLECT

John is very concerned for the well-being of the players while still cognizant of the business aspects of the team. He enjoys the respect of the rest of the medical and coaching staff and wants to maintain the strong professional relationship that he has. At the same time, he respects the players' expertise and their drive, but he knows that their long-term future can easily be in his hands, and he is most concerned about his first priority—the athletes—that are his patients. He wonders if his decision making has been affected by the pressure of the team management.

After working through the ethical decision-making process, what course of action would you suggest?

Ethical Decision-Making Worksheet

Case: _____

The Realm   Jack Glaser (1994)

Individual	Organizational/ Institutional	Societal
The good of the patient/client and focuses on rights, duties, relationships and behaviors between individuals	Good of the organization, focuses on structures and systems, which facilitate organizational or institutional goals	Concerned with the common good

The Realm _____

Rationale:

The Individual Process: James Rest (1994, 1999)

Moral Sensitivity	Moral Judgment	Moral Motivation	Moral Courage	Moral Potency (Hannah and Avolio, 2010)
Recognizing, interpreting, and framing an ethical situation	Right versus wrong actions. Generating options, selecting and applying ethical principles	Priority on ethical values over other values. Professionalism is a primary motivator for ethical behavior	Implementing the chosen ethical action, development of a plan	Includes decision making that includes moral ownership, courage, and self-efficacy

The Individual Process: _____

Rationale:

The Situation   Swisher et al. (2005) adapted from Kidder

Issue/ Problem	Dilemma	Distress	Temptation	Silence
Important values present	Two alternative courses of action: Right vs. Right decision	The right course of action is known but the clinician cannot perform it	Choice between right and wrong	Values are challenged but no one is speaking about this challenge to values

The Situation: _____

Rationale: _____

(continued on following page)

Ethical Principles and/or Standards of Ethical Conduct of the PTA (see Appendixes A and B)

Code of Ethics (Principles) for PTs	Rationale	Standards of Ethical Conduct (Standards) for PTAs	Rationale

Suggested Action:

Case Example 11

ARE YOU THE PT FOR ME?
Self-assessment to determine what is best for the patient

Every physical therapist has the obligation to do an ongoing assessment of their own professional skills and determine those aspects of PT practice that they are competent to provide safely and effectively and those that it would be in the best interest of the patient if they were referred to a PT colleague better prepared to handle their case. But even if we are well aware of our strengths and limitations, we may be challenged when we are asked to do something that we have the professional ability to do but the circumstances make us uncomfortable.

Angela was the only PT at Shady Oaks, a long-term care facility (LTC). She had been there for close to ten years and was always happy to dispel the bad press that some LTC facilities get. The nursing care was consistently good, and PT services were excellent if she did say so herself. She heard nightmare stories from some of her colleagues in other facilities about having to over or under treat patients based on priorities that seemed to be rooted in payment rather than concern for patients. In addition, the relationship between the staff, particularly nursing and rehabilitation services, was collegial and respectful. One Friday afternoon, right before Angela was ready to sign out, she was approached by Ted, the Assistant Manager of Shady Oaks, who she knew, but rarely saw or interacted with. They exchanged pleasantries and then he shared with her the reason he sought her out. He asked her if she was aware that Gwen, one of the evening nursing staff, fell in the parking lot a few days before and injured her shoulder when she landed on her arm. She stepped into a puddle, but the puddle was hiding a rather large hole in the parking lot that was not marked with any kind of warning. Ted shared with Angela that he anticipated that Gwen could be out of work for a little while to recover. Physical therapy was prescribed and based on her progress in PT the doctor will release her to return to work. Angela assumed that Ted was sharing all of this information with her so she could provide a few names of places for Gwen to go to for her PT. It had been awhile since she really thought about the orthopedic practices in the area, so she was prepared to tell Ted that she would do a little research and get back to him ... but he surprised her when he told her to expect Gwen the following morning for her first PT session at Shady Oaks. Her initial response to Ted was she had no idea how to bill workman's compensation. Shady Oaks' patients usually had Medicare and sometimes had Medicare and Medicaid. She was not sure it was even legal to treat somebody in their facility that wasn't an in-patient; they did not have an outpatient department. She managed to express that concern to Ted; he chuckled, thanked her for thinking about the bottom line but assured her it was not anything she needed to worry about, it would be taken care of.

Angela stood in the hallway watching Ted retreat back to the administrative wing, thinking to herself that the payment was probably just the tip of the iceberg. Angela did not know Gwen; they were never on the same shift, but they did lots of corresponding via memo and email regarding patients. As a colleague she of course was concerned that Gwen gets the best, and most appropriate care possible. Angela started reflecting; it had been years since she treated a patient with an acute shoulder problem— after all at Shady Oaks, they prided themselves on a great safety record ... for patients, limiting acute problems. But, it wasn't like she didn't know what to do. On the other hand, did she even have the facilities to treat a patient with an acute problem? Giving it a little bit more thought, Angela started to consider the possible ramifications of treating a person with a workman's compensation related injury "in house." Though they really did not know one another, they were colleagues, and clearly her responsibility was to her patient. Could she fulfill that responsibility when the facility is also concerned about her patient's "return to work date"? The whole situation did not seem "right" but she's a solo practitioner, and the others she usually consults with on "sticky issues" may have a different take on this situation ... like the Director of Nursing who is concerned about her employee but also concerned about staffing and having a staff member out for an extended period. The Director of Clinical Services (DCS) is another one of her sounding boards, but are they a completely neutral party, after all this accident occurred presumably as a result of negligence on the part of Shady Oaks, does the DCS have a dual role and conflicted loyalty in the situation? On the other hand, it would be kind of fun to brush up on some of those manual skills she has not used for a while. One thing she knew for certain, she had to make a decision before tomorrow morning and do so with the focus on Gwen.

CONSIDER AND REFLECT

Where Gwen receives her physical therapy services raises several questions that Angela is grappling with: Is the skill set she has the best for the patient at this time in her recovery? If she accepts Gwen as a patient and the outcome is not good where will the blame lie? Should she continue to be concerned if treating Gwen in this setting is legal or just accept the word of the administration that everything is OK. Does she have a responsibility to her colleague/patient Gwen to make sure that the proper processes are followed in the event her condition does not improve and Gwen needs more care than initially anticipated?

Angela is surprised that she is the only one that thinks there may be some inherent problems in the plan to treat a staff member for a work-related injury in an in-patient facility, and though she wasn't happy to admit it, she questioned her own skill set with regard to treating Gwen. Though she was sure she could provide adequate care ... is adequate in the best interest of the patient.

After working through the ethical decision-making process, what course of action would you suggest?

Ethical Decision-Making Worksheet

Case: _____

The Realm   Jack Glaser (1994)

Individual	Organizational/ Institutional	Societal
The good of the patient/client and focuses on rights, duties, relationships and behaviors between individuals	Good of the organization, focuses on structures and systems, which facilitate organizational or institutional goals	Concerned with the common good

(continued on following page)

The Realm: _____

Rationale:

The Individual Process   James Rest (1994, 1999)

Moral Sensitivity	Moral Judgment	Moral Motivation	Moral Courage	Moral Potency (Hannah and Avolio, 2010)
Recognizing, interpreting, and framing an ethical situation	Right vs. wrong actions. Generating options, selecting and applying ethical principles	Priority on ethical values over other values. Professionalism is a primary motivator for ethical behavior	Implementing the chosen ethical action, development of a plan	Includes decision making that includes moral ownership, courage, and self-efficacy

The Individual Process: _____

Rationale:

The Situation   Swisher et al. (2005) adapted from Kidder

Issue/ Problem	Dilemma	Distress	Temptation	Silence
Important values present	Two alternative courses of action: Right vs. Right decision	The right course of action is known but the clinician cannot perform it	Choice between right and wrong	Values are challenged but no one is speaking about this challenge to values

The Situation: _____

Rationale:

Ethical Principles and/or Standards of Ethical Conduct of the PTA (see Appendixes A and B)

Code of Ethics (Principles) for PTs	Rationale	Standards of Ethical Conduct (Standards) for PTAs	Rationale

(continued on following page)

Code of Ethics (Principles) for PTs	Rationale	Standards of Ethical Conduct (Standards) for PTAs	Rationale

Suggested Action:

Case Example 12

PROFESSIONAL DECISION MAKING ON THE LINE
The exercise of professional judgment

Every practice setting has its own innate challenges and special circumstances but regardless they all share similar professional expectations and responsibilities. The school setting is often quite different than the medical setting, but the requirements to adhere to the core values of excellence, integrity and collaboration are the same regardless of where we practice.

Gail has been a school-based physical therapist for most of her professional career. She is in a small district and treats in the elementary and the high school. She loves working with the children and watching them grow from the time they enter school at age 3 until they graduate from high school. She has been working with Melodee since she was three and now at age 9 she continues to receive PT, OT, Speech and of course classroom instruction, at home. She is medically fragile, and she cannot safely attend school. Melodee is non-verbal, and does not ambulate, as part of her Individualized Education Program (IEP) Gail has been positioning her in a standing table for a portion of the session that she shares with the teacher in an attempt to improve her attention during the session. Gail was planning on bringing this particular aspect of the program up at the next IEP meeting as the time to get Melodee into her orthoses for standing seems to be far more than the benefit gained from the activity. On Wednesday Gail arrives for her regularly scheduled PT session and is surprised to find that Melodee is in a nightgown and not dressed as she normally is for school. Her mom explains that Melodee was all out of sorts starting Friday evening and appeared to be in pain when her left leg was touched. They contacted the doctor, and she suggested taking Melodee to the ER for an X-ray which revealed a left femur fracture. It was a clean fracture, so they decided not to cast it but rather to immobilize it, using a soft splint to protect the site. Melodee saw the orthopedist on Monday who concurred it did not need to be set and sent a note for "PT and OT to continue, avoid any aggressive movement of the left leg." Gail was concerned as this was Melodee's second fracture this year and for both there wasn't a precipitating incident noted. This type of spontaneous fracture is of concern indicating underlying medical issues. Gail was happy to hear that apparently the Orthopedist was concerned as well referring Melodee to the endocrinologist for an evaluation. The appointment was several weeks off so there was going to be little change in the plan of care until that visit occurred. Gail attempted to reposition Melodee and began the range of motion for the right leg, but it was apparent that Melodee was very uncomfortable. Not wanting to get Melodee any more upset before the teacher arrived for the rest of the session Gail stopped any lower extremity treatment and position changes, just attempting to find a position that would be functional for the "school session." At the next visit on Friday Gail was hoping that the discomfort diminished, and she would be able to do more with Melodee but unfortunately laying in bed for almost a week it seemed like almost every movement made her uncomfortable. With the endocrinologist consult over a month away and Melodee unable to cooperate much with treatment Gail decides the appropriate course of action is to put Melodee on hold until the leg heals, and she has had the consult so they can determine where this tendency to fracture is coming from and how to decrease the risk of her fracturing again. She also justifies this plan as her treatment at this point is completely medically based. She cannot get Melodee into a position that supports the educational plan, so she is not addressing any school-based goals that are part of the IEP. She sends a quick email to the case manager outlining her plan to hold on treatment and readjusts her schedule accordingly. She is surprised when the case manager comes back to her and says that Melodee should not be placed on hold, as long as the Doctor says it is ok to treat, she does not need to stop providing services. The case manager reminds Gail that the treatment plan is in the IEP and that is a legal requirement that she has to continue to provide treatment. Gail understands the perspective of the case manager and also appreciates that the physician probably does not have a very good understanding of the nature of rehab services provided in the school setting and the need for educational relevance for the plan to be school-based. But Gail is concerned, she does know that the plan in place for Melodee is not consistent with the intent of the IEP and she does not feel she should continue to treat for that reason, as well as she feels that her continuing to treat is not helping Melodee and could potentially be harmful. Just where is the line between professional judgment and professional requirements?

CONSIDER AND REFLECT

It is not uncommon regardless of setting to be caught in a situation where we know what is best based on our professional judgment, however there are conflicting obligations that we have to acknowledge that impact our decision making. Ultimately the responsibility for taking action is ours as "no action" is a default action, and often not an acceptable one.

After working through the ethical decision-making process, what course of action would you suggest?

Ethical Decision-Making Worksheet

Case: _____

The Realm

Jack Glaser (1994)

Individual	Organizational/Institutional	Societal
The good of the patient/client and focuses on rights, duties, relationships and behaviors between individuals	Good of the organization, focuses on structures and systems, which facilitate organizational or institutional goals	Concerned with the common good

The Realm _____

Rationale:

(continued on following page)

The Individual Process: James Rest (1994, 1999)

Moral Sensitivity	Moral Judgment	Moral Motivation	Moral Courage	Moral Potency (Hannah and Avolio, 2010)
Recognizing, interpreting, and framing an ethical situation	Right versus wrong actions. Generating options, selecting and applying ethical principles	Priority on ethical values over other values. Professionalism is a primary motivator for ethical behavior	Implementing the chosen ethical action, development of a plan	Includes decision making that includes moral ownership, courage, and self-efficacy

The Individual Process: _____

Rationale:

The Situation   Swisher et al. (2005) adapted from Kidder

Issue/ Problem	Dilemma	Distress	Temptation	Silence
Important values present	Two alternative courses of action: Right vs. Right decision	The right course of action is known but the clinician cannot perform it	Choice between right and wrong	Values are challenged but no one is speaking about this challenge to values

The Situation: _____

Rationale: _____

Ethical Principles and/or Standards of Ethical Conduct of the PTA (see Appendixes A and B)

Code of Ethics (Principles) for PTs	Rationale	Standards of Ethical Conduct (Standards) for PTAs	Rationale

(continued on following page)

Code of Ethics (Principles) for PTs	Rationale	Standards of Ethical Conduct (Standards) for PTAs	Rationale

Suggested Action:

CHAPTER 14

Professional Relationships

Physical therapists (PTs) are an integral part of the healthcare team. While all PTs recognize that they are ultimately responsible for their actions, PTs never practice in isolation. Professional relationships between therapists and PT assistants and other healthcare providers and healthcare administrators are crucial to the safe and effective delivery of healthcare. Working as part of a team requires mutual respect and trust, two virtues that are common to all healthcare providers. As part of professional training students are often required to work in a group to become accustomed to participating in effective group process. These groups are in an intra-professional setting, consisting of PTs and PTAs. Education particularly in a large academic medical center environment allows for exposure to other professionals, opportunities to engage in interprofessional education (IPE) and ultimately inter-professional practice (IPP). Professional relationships require good communication and a willingness to listen, absorb, and consider other viewpoints.

Professionals interact with one another on many different levels. This provides opportunities to serve as mentors, or act as a supervisor or a supervisee, or some-times both simultaneously. Teamwork requires a basic understanding of what our colleagues contribute to patient care so we can complement one another. Team communication is complicated, and it requires that every professional be willing to enter into a relationship of mutual respect for the benefit of the patient. The cases in this section look at professional relationships from very different perspectives; they share in common challenges to the very virtues that are part of professional practice.

Joint Moves	**Respect for interprofessional practice**
An Acute Cold Shoulder	**Destructive professional relationship**
Homesick	**Professional power gradient abuse**

Case Example 13

JOINT MOVES
Respect for interprofessional practice

In most cases, our relationship as physical therapists to our colleagues in other healthcare disciplines is excellent. Sometimes, however, situations arise that place us in the uncomfortable position of balancing, on the one hand, our fiduciary obligation and concern for our patient, and, on the other hand, our professional respect for healthcare colleagues who also are serving that patient. Consider the following scenario.

Jim has been a solo private practitioner for more than twenty years. While he practices in a small town, it is located within a large metropolitan area, so his patients and clients have many choices for physical therapy. Jim takes pride in the fact that he has many longtime patrons from larger towns and cities in the area. He has established strong relationships with many area physicians, to whom he refers patients and who, likewise, refer their patients to him.

Mitch is a sixty-two-year-old construction worker and avid "weekend warrior" who has come to Jim for various physical issues over the years related to his strenuous job and hard-driving recreational pursuits. Mitch's hip has been wearing down for some time, and Jim has counseled the eventual need for replacement surgery. After resisting the idea for months, during a physical therapy session after a weekend of escalating pain Mitch concedes that he sees the wisdom in having the medical procedure.

It is Jim's custom to give his patients a few options among the physicians with whom he regularly works. He gives Mitch the names of three surgeons, all of whom he wholeheartedly recommends. Noting that Mitch's company insurance covers "prehabilitation" in the weeks immediately preceding such surgery, Jim further recommends that he and Mitch work together to get him as strong as possible for the hip-replacement procedure and postsurgery physical therapy.

Mitch readily agrees to prehab. Jim is a bit surprised when Mitch selects for the surgery a physician who isn't among those Jim had recommended—saying a coworker told him "this guy is really good"—but Jim certainly respects Mitch's right to make his own decisions. Jim is unfamiliar with the physician, but is determined, as always, to help his patient get into the best possible shape for surgery and postsurgery physical therapy.

Two weeks after his final presurgery physical therapy session—after surgery and a brief stint in rehab—Mitch returns to Jim's clinic. Although Mitch seems optimistic and clearly is excited about the prospect of getting back to work soon, Jim is concerned to note, during the course of his evaluation, that Mitch's surgical scar is significantly more extensive than those he has seen in many years. Jim is also discomfited by the fact that the prosthesis had dislocated shortly after surgery and had to be refitted.

Still, dislocations do happen on occasion, Jim knows. What's most important to Jim is that Mitch is well-versed in the precautions he's been instructed to observe to prevent another dislocation. I'm going to be a good patient and get back to business," Mitch says.

Jim schedules Mitch's next appointment for later that week, but he is surprised first thing the next morning to find Doris, Mitch's wife, in the waiting room and looking frantic. She reports that Mitch is outside in the car, is in a lot of pain, and that they believe the new hip popped out again an hour earlier. Can Jim please take a look?

Jim helps Mitch inside and immediately sees that, sure enough, the hip once again has dislocated. "I swear, I did everything the doc said!" Mitch exclaims. "I just heard a pop when I stood up. So, is there something you can do to help me out?"

"I'm sorry, but you need to go to the emergency room," Jim responds. Mitch is disappointed, but he agrees. Jim helps Mitch back to his car and Doris takes the wheel to drive her husband to the hospital.

It's another two weeks and a surgical repair procedure later before Jim sees Mitch again. "The doc says it must've been something I did or you did," Mitch reports. "I'm sure it wasn't you, so I'm thinking I must not have been careful enough." While Jim is gratified by Mitch's faith in him, he feels certain that his patient in no way contributed to his current circumstance.

"Now that you've had this second procedure, the worst should be behind you," Jim tells Mitch. "Still, you might want to get another medical opinion, given the difficulties you've had." He suggests that Jim contact one of the physicians whose name he'd given Mitch initially. While Jim doesn't want to give an impression of impugning the competence of Mitch's surgeon, rarely do any of Jim's patients experience *any* significant setbacks after joint replacement surgery, let alone two postsurgical incidents. Thus, Jim feels strongly that Mitch would benefit from the opinion of a second surgeon.

To Jim's dismay, however, Mitch replies, "I'm done with doctors and procedures! I'll see you bright and early Monday morning for physical therapy. It's high time for me to get back to work!"

But Mitch is a no-show Monday morning. Concerned by his absence, Jim calls Mitch's house but gets the answering machine. About an hour later, a distressed Doris calls from the hospital to report that Mitch is in the ER because the new hip again has dislocated. Jim expresses his concern and sympathy and asks Doris to keep him apprised of further developments.

After he puts the phone down, Jim sits at his desk and ponders the situation. Surely *now* Mitch will consult with another physician. But what if he doesn't? What if Mitch remains convinced that he's somehow to blame for the dislocations—or comes to believe, based on what his physician had said, that physical therapy has played a role in the setbacks? If Mitch declines to seek a second opinion, should Jim simply "cut bait" and terminate his relationship with Mitch, he wonders. Should he suggest that Mitch see a different PT?

CONSIDER AND REFLECT

Jim wants what is best for his patient, but if Mitch should be unwilling to take his advice, there could be implications for Jim's practice, reputation, and, perhaps, his livelihood. Poor surgical outcomes certainly will affect Jim's ability to effectively progress Mitch, reflecting poorly on the perceived quality of Jim's care. Furthermore, the seeds of doubt the physician has sewn about Jim's work could leave Jim open to future litigation.

Jim knows the frequent dislocations may have a nonsurgical cause, and he doesn't wish to give the appearance of questioning that aspect of the physician's work. Jim does feel, however, that Mitch would benefit from the opinion of a physician who's willing to explore other causes, rather than simply blaming the patient or the PT.

Jim believes a second opinion is necessary to determine what is causing recurrent dislocations that are adversely affecting Mitch's recovery and livelihood, as well as Jim's ability to protect Mitch from reinjury and facilitate his recovery. Should Mitch continue to decline this option, Jim worries about his patient's physical well-being and his own reputation and practice. He does not wish, however, to be seen as, or gain a reputation among referring physicians for discrediting the work or decision making of another medical professional.

After working through the ethical decision-making process, what course of action would you suggest?

Ethical Decision-Making Worksheet

Case: _____

The Realm   Jack Glaser (1994)

Individual	Organizational/ Institutional	Societal
The good of the patient/ client and focuses on rights, duties, relationships, and behaviors between individuals	Good of the organization, focuses on structures and systems, which facilitate organizational or institutional goals	Concerned with the common good

The Realm: _____

Rationale:

(continued on following page)

The Individual Process

James Rest (1994, 1999)

Moral Sensitivity	Moral Judgment	Moral Motivation	Moral Courage	Moral Potency (Hannah and Avolio, 2010)
Recognizing, interpreting, and framing an ethical situation	Right vs. wrong actions. Generating options, selecting and applying ethical principles	Priority on ethical values over other values. Professionalism is a primary motivator for ethical behavior	Implementing the chosen ethical action, development of a plan	Includes decision making that includes moral ownership, courage, and self-efficacy

The Individual Process: _____

Rationale:

The Situation

Swisher et al. (2005) adapted from Kidder

Issue/ Problem	Dilemma	Distress	Temptation	Silence
Important values present	Two alternative courses of action: Right vs. Right decision	The right course of action is known but the clinician cannot perform it	Choice between right and wrong	Values are challenged but no one is speaking about this challenge to values

The Situation: _____

Rationale:

Ethical Principles and/or Standards of Ethical Conduct of the PTA (see Appendixes A and B)

Code of Ethics (Principles) for PTs	Rationale	Standards of Ethical Conduct (Standards) for PTAs	Rationale

(continued on following page)

Code of Ethics (Principles) for PTs	Rationale	Standards of Ethical Conduct (Standards) for PTAs	Rationale

Suggested Action:

Case Example 14

AN ACUTE COLD SHOULDER
Destructive professional relationship

Among the many joys of being a physical therapist (PT) or physical therapist assistant (PTA) are the relationships we form with our colleagues, which not only enrich us personally, but which also make us better at what we do, as we all work together on behalf of the patients and clients we serve. What happens, though, when the colleagues to whom we turn for professional guidance and interpersonal collegiality turn their backs on us rather than extending their hand?

Gloria graduated from a master's level PT education program more than twenty years ago. She worked at a hospital for two years, until her first child was born, and continued to work there part-time until she gave birth to a second child a year later. At that point, she opted to stay home to raise her children. Five years later, she and her husband had a third child.

She loved working in acute care, and she always planned to return to work. For that reason, she met all the requirements to maintain her license during her extended hiatus from physical therapy, even through the upheaval of several relocations around the state. Gloria also retained her APTA membership in order to keep up with the latest developments in practice and research.

With her two oldest children in college and the youngest now in high school, she decides the time is right to return to the work she'd so enjoyed earlier in her life. She eagerly starts researching local employers and scanning job listings. She uses a Physical Therapy Practice Review Tool to compare her knowledge, skills, and abilities against those of current entry-level practitioners, and feels gratified when its "candidate feedback report" assesses her overall performance as "sufficiently qualified" (as opposed to "needs improvement"). This affirmation emboldens her to apply for an open position at City General Hospital. The post particularly appeals to her because it entails working only one weekend per month. With her youngest child still in high school and a variety of volunteer obligations she has taken on over the years, she prefers to dip a toe back into the waters of PT work rather than immerse herself right off the bat. While she feels confident in her abilities, she also wants to be certain she still enjoys working in the hospital setting.

Gloria is thrilled when she gets the job. She had learned during the interview process that all the PTs with whom she'll be working are seasoned veterans. She looks forward to their mentoring assistance, and to experiencing the professional camaraderie she has missed during her years away from the workplace.

Her supervisor, Patty, has set up a weeklong orientation to get Gloria started. She's told that she'll be shadowing a PT named Mildred. The assignment initially excites Gloria, because it's quickly apparent that Mildred knows not only the ropes, but seemingly everyone at the hospital, regardless of their position, department, or healthcare discipline. Gloria is sure to feel not only well-schooled but also well-connected by week's end, she believes.

Mildred does prove to be an excellent instructor of the duties that Gloria will be assuming, and of the ins and outs of getting things done at City General. Gloria is considerably less pleased, however, with the way Mildred is introducing her around the hospital. She typically describes Gloria to other PTs and staff as either a "new" or an "inexperienced" therapist who's "really going to need your help, because she's been a stay-at-home mom for 20 years." Gloria can't tell if Mildred is trying to be help-ful but going about it in an insensitive way, or if she genuinely questions Gloria's abilities. Gloria frequently interjects such corrective comments as, "I have acute care experience" and "I've never let my license lapse," but Mildred's introductions don't change.

Furthermore, Gloria can't seem to ask a simple question without provoking impatience or, on occasion, outright eye-rolling from Mildred. Gloria deems this not only as unprofessional behavior, but also as utterly unfair, given that her queries have nothing to do with her competence and everything to do with the simple fact that she is new on the job.

Still, as the week progresses and Gloria is granted more and more autonomy, she knows she has made the right decision by returning to work. She loves the hospital setting and her interactions with patients. Whatever Mildred's problem with her might be, Mildred won't be there when Gloria begins her weekend shifts. On Friday afternoon, she seeks the veteran PT out to thank her for her help. Mildred and two other PTs are in the midst of discussing an after-hours happy hour. Mildred responds to Gloria's thanks with a quick, "You bet, hon," then resumes her conversation with the other PTs. Gloria is a bit disappointed that no one invites her to come along. She reasons, however, that they probably assume she'd rather go straight home at the end of her busy orientation week.

The plan is for Gloria initially to work at City General every other weekend, so she quickly can gain experience and establish an on-the-job "rhythm," then cut back to her standing schedule of a single weekend per month. Again, Gloria enjoys all the physical therapy-related aspects of her job, but she finds many of Mildred's behaviors and mannerisms reflected in the weekend-shift PTs with whom she now works. Like Mildred, they almost uniformly have little patience with her questions. One of them recently even exclaimed with exasperation, "Where have you been? Oh, that's right!"—suggesting that Gloria is insufficiently knowledgeable about current practice. (In fact, however, in many instances Gloria believes she is better versed in the latest literature than are her colleagues.)

Even in the cafeteria, the other PTs—and the nurses with whom they socialize—are so unwelcoming toward her that Gloria generally eats by herself. The only exception is a PT named Marie who sometimes subs on weekends. She advises Gloria, "Don't let the mean girls get to you. It takes a while to earn their respect. You just need to tough it out."

Gloria considers Marie's words. She tries to be upbeat in her dealings with her colleagues, but as the months go on, not only does the dismissive treatment continue, but Gloria sometimes is reprimanded for poor time management when equipment she needs is unavailable at the time when she plans to use it with patients—even though she has announced in advance that she'll be requiring it. Is it just her imagination, or are her colleagues sometimes trying to sabotage her treatment sessions?

One night—about six months into the job, and two months after she has dropped down to one weekend a month—she joins her son for a weeknight program sponsored by the high school guidance department. The main focus is on college preparation, but there is a segment on something that is identified as a "too-often underappreciated deterrent" to optimal academic performance and student socialization. That deterrent is bullying. As the speaker describes the phenomenon of bullying—what it looks like and the effects it can have—Gloria feels as if he is talking directly to her about what she has been enduring at City General.

The connection is revelatory. Gloria had never really thought of bullying in an adult, let alone a workplace, context. But now she starts putting the pieces together as she considers the scene at City General: A veteran, insular staff. Overheard references to "short-timers" who "couldn't last here." Marie's comment about the "mean girls." Gloria truly loves the patient-care aspects of her job and doesn't want to leave. The dismissiveness and ostracism are wearing on her, however—and they may be the cause of those "time-management issues" that are affecting her ability to optimally perform her duties.

Is bullying among adults, Gloria wonders, really a "thing"? Is she perhaps being too thin-skinned about a form of professional hazing that ultimately might make her a stronger—even a better—PT? At any rate, what recourse does she have? Can her supervisor, Patty, possibly be unaware of this hostile work environment toward newcomers? Should Gloria broach the subject with her, will Patty be sympathetic? If she is, what actions might Patty take to change things for the better?

Will she ultimately gain from stirring up a hornet's nest, Gloria wonders, or simply get multiply stung?

CONSIDER AND REFLECT

It is not uncommon for adults to overlook the classic signs of bullying and fail to recognize their applicability to adult situations. This scenario fits the definition invoked by the Workplace Bullying Institute and cited on its website (www.workplacebullying.org). The institute defines workplace bullying as "repeated, health-harming mistreatment of one or more persons by one or more perpetrators." It is, furthermore, "abusive conduct that is threatening, humiliating, or intimidating, and can result in workplace interference/sabotage." Workplace bullying, the institute holds, is a cousin of domestic violence in which "the abuser is on the payroll."

Bullying among adults and in the workplace goes unreported and unnoticed for the most part. Most adults are either embarrassed to mention it or feel they really do not have any recourse and do not want to provide additional ammunition for their tormentors. While not reported it is still quite real (Oeffner, 2014).

After working through the ethical decision-making process, what course of action would you suggest?

Ethical Decision-Making Worksheet

Case: _____

The Realm   Jack Glaser (1994)

Individual	Organizational/ Institutional	Societal
The good of the patient/client and focuses on rights, duties, relationships, and behaviors between individuals	Good of the organization, focuses on structures and systems, which facilitate organizational or institutional goals	Concerned with the common good

(continued on following page)

The Realm: _____

Rationale:

The Individual Process   James Rest (1994, 1999)

Moral Sensitivity	Moral Judgment	Moral Motivation	Moral Courage	Moral Potency (Hannah and Avolio, 2010)
Recognizing, interpreting, and framing an ethical situation	Right vs. wrong actions. Generating options, selecting and applying ethical principles	Priority on ethical values over other values. Professionalism is a primary motivator for ethical behavior	Implementing the chosen ethical action, development of a plan	Includes decision making that includes moral ownership, courage, and self-efficacy

The Individual Process: _____

Rationale:

The Situation: Swisher et al. (2005) adapted from Kidder

Issue/ Problem	Dilemma	Distress	Temptation	Silence
Important values present	Two alternative courses of action: Right vs. Right decision	The right course of action is known but the clinician cannot perform it	Choice between right and wrong	Values are challenged but no one is speaking about this challenge to values

The Situation: _____

Rationale:

Ethical Principles and/or Standards of Ethical Conduct of the PTA (see Appendixes A and B)

Code of Ethics (Principles) for PTs	Rationale	Standards of Ethical Conduct (Standards) for PTAs	Rationale

(continued on following page)

Code of Ethics (Principles) for PTs	Rationale	Standards of Ethical Conduct (Standards) for PTAs	Rationale

Suggested Action:

Case Example 15

Physical therapists have a well-deserved reputation worldwide as caring individuals who are dedicated to providing optimal patient and client care. Every profession has its exceptions, however. In the following scenario, a newcomer to this country has the misfortune to be paired with one such practitioner.

HOMESICK
Professional power gradient abuse

Vern has worked for five years as a licensed physical therapist (PT) in his home country, where he was a respected supervisor at a subacute care facility. But his longtime dream is to practice in the United States, so he initiates the long and involved process of organizing his paperwork, getting his credentials evaluated, qualifying and studying for the National Physical Therapy Examination (NPTE), and applying for an H-1B visa. Obtaining the latter requires that he has "an employer–employee relationship with the petitioning U.S. employer."

It's a tedious process, but the recruiter with whom Vern works has been invaluable in guiding the PT through the various steps and all the red tape. It takes him two tries, but a determined Vern passes the NPTE and is excited to have several employment options from which to choose. The recruiter assures him that all the facilities are outstanding, and officials at each have reviewed his credentials and are eager to add him to their care team.

Vern selects Tall Oaks Restorative Care, a subacute facility located in the rural South. The practice setting will be familiar, he reasons, and from what he's read, the climate and pace of life will be reminiscent of home.

Vern eagerly prepares himself for his first day at Tall Oaks—joining APTA, studying the state practice act and passing the jurisprudence exam, and reviewing hot issues, as well as ethics and professionalism in the U.S. profession, by studying materials posted or linked to APTA's website.

Finally, the big day arrives. Vern has been in town for a couple of weeks—long enough to secure an apartment, choose a coffee shop, and locate the nearest laundromat. He can barely contain his enthusiasm as he walks through the door of his new workplace. Everyone seems very friendly and happy to have him onboard. Vern spends much of the morning filling out paperwork, with the help of his recruiter via cellphone. Then he is brought to the physical therapy department, where he is introduced to Claire—the employer of the "employer–employee relationship" that is referenced on Vern's H-1B visa.

Like everyone else he has met at Tall Oaks, Claire seems delighted by Vern's arrival on the scene. She explains that in addition to supervising physical therapy at the facility, she owns a company that contracts services to Tall Oaks and a few other subacute facilities in the area. "I've found Tall Oaks to be the most difficult to staff," she says, "which is why you're here."

Vern isn't sure whether to take that as a compliment or simply as a sigh of relief on Claire's part—especially when she informs him that she and he are the only PTs at Tall Oaks—a ninety-bed facility with thirty-subacute beds. "We also have an awesome aide named Mark to help us out," Claire hastens to add.

Vern is wondering how two PTs possibly can manage such a large caseload and what his responsibilities will be. As if reading his mind, Claire says, "Let's discuss how this all will work over a nice lunch at a family restaurant down the street."

The food at the restaurant is good, and Vern is starting to feel a little more relaxed. But suddenly he's jolted by a statement Claire makes. "Your predecessor didn't stay long," she says, "so you can probably imagine why I jumped at the chance to hire a foreigner who'll be thankful just to have a good job in this country." Claire is smiling as she says this, but Vern isn't at all sure she's joking. He's even less certain when, during the course of the next half hour, Claire brings the conversation back several times to the fact that she and he are "joined at the hip" by the requirements of his visa.

When they return to Tall Oaks, Vern meets Mark, who's very friendly but also is quite busy, supervising four patients who are working out in the gym. After a few minutes he excuses himself, saying, "I need to go get the rest of the 1 o'clock patients." Vern is confused. The rest?

Who's responsible for the patients already in the gym? Who's expected to treat the new patients? Which patients are his, and which are Claire's? What role, precisely, is Mark playing with physical therapy patients at Tall Oaks?

Just then, Claire emerges from her office and says, "Isn't Mark great?" She hands Vern a notebook and says she's off to a meeting. "Check the charts if you have any questions," she calls over her shoulder as she exits the room. "You guys be good! I'll see you in a few hours."

Mark returns with two additional patients. He asks them to "hold tight" for a few minutes, starts working with a couple of the other patients in the gym, and motions for Vern to come jump in. Vern is thoroughly disoriented. He knows from his studies that, while physical therapist assistants (PTAs) in the United States have some latitude in working with patients under the supervision of a PT, the duties an aide can legally perform are quite limited. Still, Vern has patients to treat. Many patients. He gets busy applying his skills.

Around 5 pm, Claire returns, explaining that her meeting ran long, and she had to pick up her teenage daughter from school afterward and drive her to the pool.

"Well, I'm glad you're back, because I have a lot of questions for you," Vern says.

"I'll bet you do!" Claire breezily responds. "Tell you what—go ahead and complete your patient notes. Don't worry about billing; that's my job. Get yourself some well-deserved rest tonight and we'll pick up this discussion in the morning, because I've got to scoot on home now. Okay?"

With that, she's gone. Mark can see that Vern's facial expression begs the question, "What just happened here?" Mark chuckles and says, "The PT before you called Claire 'greased lightning.' She's all about movement—except when it comes to patient care."

Vern sleeps poorly that night and arrives at Tall Oaks the next morning determined to get answers. Claire, however, has stayed home—reportedly to tend to her sick 6-year-old daughter. Vern's workload is even more intense than it had been on his first day. He's confident in his abilities as a PT and does the best he can under the circumstances. Mark is helpful, but he obviously is performing beyond his scope of work as an aide, and he lacks the knowledge and training of a PT or PTA. Meanwhile, the paperwork, on which Vern has received no guidance, continues to vex him.

Claire returns the next morning. Vern corrals her as soon as she has settled into her office. She appears calm and says she'll be happy to answer any question he has.

Vern notes that there are far more patients than there are PTs at Tall Oaks. "We do the best we can," Claire says. "My philosophy is quality, not quantity of minutes. Anyway, this isn't unusual in the US. Our health care system's overburdened."

Vern notes that Mark, an aide, seems to be carrying a full patient case-load, as if he were a PT. How can that be? "I trained Mark well," Claire responds, "but believe me, I keep a close eye on everything he does. An advanced degree isn't everything, you know. Mark has great instincts. At any rate, it's my business how I use him."

Vern then asks Claire about the "verification of treatment" document—the one that describes services performed and attests that all were billed correctly. Vern has not been signing the documents because he hasn't seen any billing, and thus has no way of knowing whether it is correct. "You need to sign those documents and include your license number, the same way you sign your notes," Claire says. "Let me worry about the billing. All you need to know is that I'm making sure we get paid, so that we don't need to lay off anyone."

Is Vern hearing what he thinks he's hearing? Is Claire threatening his job? Any doubt about that is dispelled when Claire again returns to the subject of their employer–employee relationship. The unmistakable message is that, were he to lose his job at Tall Oaks, the H-1B visa agreement would be compromised.

As if Vern doesn't already feel sufficiently bullied by Claire, she adds, "You know, there's a noncompete clause in the agreement with your recruiter. That means you can't be placed with another employer if you should leave here in less than a year. And you know what that would mean to your stay in the US," she says. "No job, no visa."

Vern is speechless. Claire wraps up the discussion. "Another busy day in paradise!" she says in a light tone. "Look," she adds. "Don't get me wrong. I'm happy to have you here. You seem very conscientious—and, I have to say, more competent than I'd dared hope you'd be, coming from another country. You can make this easy for yourself or you can make it hard. Personally, I'm optimistic that we can make this work, help our patients, and make the best of the situation. What do you say?"

Vern cannot say what he's really thinking, which is that "helping patients" seems far from Claire's priorities. There clearly are bigger issues at play here than Vern's own employment and visa status. Making it "easy on himself," by Claire's definition, will ill-serve patients—and will deal Vern's personal integrity a crippling blow.

CONSIDER AND REFLECT

Claire clearly is taking advantage of Vern. He has invested great time, money, and resources in his decision to practice in the United States, but he is at her mercy—as she pointedly highlights. These aggressive actions cause or threaten to cause improper use of PT resources, and compromise best practice. Claire seems to fear no consequences for her behavior, but for Vern the stakes are high: losing his job, visa, and license on the one hand, or forfeiting his ethical and professional integrity on the other.

After working through the ethical decision-making process, what course of action would you suggest?

Ethical Decision-Making Worksheet

Case: _____

The Realm

Jack Glaser (1994)

Individual	Organizational/ Institutional	Societal
The good of the patient/ client and focuses on rights, duties, relationships, and behaviors between individuals	Good of the organization, focuses on structures and systems, which facilitate organizational or institutional goals	Concerned with the common good

The Realm: _____

Rationale:

The Individual Process

James Rest (1994, 1999)

Moral Sensitivity	Moral Judgment	Moral Motivation	Moral Courage	Moral Potency (Hannah and Avolio, 2010)
Recognizing, interpreting, and framing an ethical situation	Right vs. wrong actions. Generating options, selecting and applying ethical principles	Priority on ethical values over other values. Professionalism is a primary motivator for ethical behavior	Implementing the chosen ethical action, development of a plan	Includes decision making that includes moral ownership, courage, and self-efficacy

The Individual Process: _____

Rationale:

(continued on following page)

The Situation
Swisher et al. (2005) adapted from Kidder

Issue/ Problem	Dilemma	Distress	Temptation	Silence
Important values present	Two alternative courses of action: Right vs. Right decision	The right course of action is known but the clinician cannot perform it	Choice between right and wrong	Values are challenged but no one is speaking about this challenge to values

The Situation: _____

Rationale:

Ethical Principles and/or Standards of Ethical Conduct of the PTA (see Appendixes A and B)

Code of Ethics (Principles) for PTs	Rationale	Standards of Ethical Conduct (Standards) for PTAs	Rationale

Suggested Action:

Case Example 16

UNWELCOME NOTICE
Professional disrespect

Kenny has been at the Middlebury office of InMotion PT for four years. Joining the established staff at Middlebury straight out of school he is grateful to the company for their support and mentoring during that time. He achieved his OCS last year and continues to hone his skills surrounded by, as he calls them "the gurus" of manual therapy. The growth of his clinical skills has not been the only change over the past few years. He married his College sweetheart, Kendra, two years ago and they are ecstatic to be expecting their first child in just a few months. The staff, most many years his senior, kid him about how he is settling down and becoming kind of "boring" like them. He just chuckles, thinking they are anything but boring, they may be married and have kids, but they are up for an adventure anytime and the talk in the office is often about the next Iron Man or training for the next 10K. His colleagues are not short on advice when he informs them on Monday that he and Kendra put a bid on a house, it was accepted and on top of everything else verifying his new "adult status" he was going to have a mortgage. Mary, the site coordinator was particularly interested in Kenny's new home inquiring how soon they planned to move and pointing out to him that the new house, while located in a lovely suburban area of the county was quite a bit further away from the Middlebury office than his current apartment and going with the traffic in both directions. Kenny appreciating her observation and concern shared with her that he and Kendra had discussed that a lot and decided that since she worked from home he could extend his commute a bit, she would be able to manage the home front, and it was exactly where they wanted to raise a family. Mary raised the question again the next day, this time sharing with Kenny how many times she changed positions to better meet the needs of her family as they were younger. Kenny was getting concerned, was she afraid he could not manage the commute and would leave InMotion PT? Or was she trying to hint to him that she did not feel he would be able to manage a new baby, a long commute, and his long hours at the office. A few days later Mary asked Kenny to stick around as the office closed that evening "to talk." Kenny wondered if this was related in some way to their discussion earlier in the week and was anxious for the last patient to finish up so he could sit down with Mary and assure her that he was up to the task of managing his new lifestyle and had no intention of leaving InMotion PT. Mary was very direct, starting with just how pleased they have been with Kenny's work and how they all take pride in how he has grown as a clinician, but they actually needed him to step up and take on a new challenge for the company. Kenny was surprised, this is not at all what he was expecting. InMotion was the biggest PT provider in the tricounty area, but Kenny was really only aware of The Middlebury office. With seven PTs and two PTAs it was the flagship of the six offices in the company. Mary shared with him that the Parkland office just learned of the retirement of Lydia a PT that had been with the company since it started and the owners of InMotion in light of recent events, felt the offices were in need of some "rebalancing" and since he was so well thought of that he could bring several things to the Parkland office. Kenny, not quite sure, of exactly what those things were ... looked a little confused. Mary offered some clarification, "To be perfectly frank we need a little diversity in Parkland. There are four positions, 3 PT and 1 PTA. All are women and all are over 50 and none of them are clinical specialists. You ring the bell on three counts, and it will be a great learning experience for you, not to mention Parkland is in your county not more than 20 minutes from your new home. I don't know about you but I think 'all the stars are aligning on this one.'"

Kenny could not wait until tomorrow, on his way home he called Barry his InMotion mentor to get his take on the "move." Apparently, Kenny was the last to know of the option to relocate afforded him as Barry seemed fully aware and on board with providing him support to make this next career move offering to continue to mentor Kenny no matter where he practiced. It all happened very quickly. Kenny took a week off to move into his new house and the following Monday showed up to Parkland excited to meet his new coworkers and patients. It did not take long for Kenny to realize, though his new coworkers were a little older, and none were clinical specialists they were very seasoned and effective clinicians, and he was in an environment that he would continue to learn and grow, and 20 minutes from home and no highway driving was another nice perk. What Kenny did not expect was what started to unfold over the next few days. Marge, the clinic director took great pleasure in introducing Kenny to his patients, to all patients as "our new eye candy" exclaiming in her booming voice things like, "Isn't he a sight to behold, just adorable, best new decorating job we have had in years." Kenny tried to quickly regain his professional demeanor after one of these ebullient introductions, but he often found it difficult. His coworkers were most welcoming as they said, "treating him like one of the girls" but he found that the office chatter that included him, was often very personal and uncomfortable for him. Kenny had absolutely no clinical issues with Parkland. His colleagues were as eager to teach him as to learn from him, but their comments about his physique, his hair, and his eyes, did embarrass and distract him. Marge would often call across the room to a patient, "I bet if you were 20 years younger you would jump at the chance to rehab that knee so you could chase Kenny around the building." Several times Kenny mentioned to Marge that while he appreciated the intent of the comments they were distracting and Marge usually responded with a booming laugh, an apology and was right back at it the next time the opportunity arose.

Following an all staff meeting one evening at the Middlebury office, Kenny asked Barry to stay a minute to chat. Barry always eager to engage in a clinical query from his young mentee was happy to oblige. Kenny shared with Barry some of the comments Marge and occasionally his other co workers made. Barry could see how uncomfortable Kenny was but had little to offer to him. He pointed out that Marge meant absolutely no harm. She was ecstatic to have Kenny at Parkland, she respected his clinical expertise and his willingness to learn. Barry knew it was just the way Marge spoke and interacted, she called herself an "ole crusty barnacle and meant no harm by her language and comments." The younger man still looked very concerned when Barry turned to him and said, "Look, just brush off the comments and the uncomfortable watercooler talk." You know Kenny, guys are not supposed to notice that kind of stuff, just buck up and let the comments roll off your back, after all do you really want to report a middle age woman for complimenting you?

CONSIDER AND REFLECT

Have you found yourself in a situation in which you experienced uncomfortable conversation either directed at you or to a colleague? Did it impact patient care? If so, how did you react? Is taking some sort of action always appropriate in such situations? What should you do when your concerns are not taken seriously and you do not feel comfortable in the workplace?

After working through the ethical decision-making process, what course of action would you suggest?

Ethical Decision Making Worksheet

Case: _____

The Realm   Jack Glaser (1994)

Individual	Organizational/ Institutional	Societal
The good of the patient/client and focuses on rights, duties, relationships and behaviors between individuals	Good of the organization, focuses on structures and systems, which facilitate organizational or institutional goals	Concerned with the common good

(continued on following page)

The Realm _____

Rationale:

The Individual Process: James Rest (1994, 1999)

Moral Sensitivity	Moral Judgment	Moral Motivation	Moral Courage	Moral Potency (Hannah and Avolio, 2010)
Recognizing, interpreting, and framing an ethical situation	Right versus wrong actions. Generating options, selecting and applying ethical principles	Priority on ethical values over other values. Professionalism is a primary motivator for ethical behavior	Implementing the chosen ethical action, development of a plan	Includes decision making that includes moral ownership, courage, and self-efficacy

The Individual Process: _____

Rationale:

The Situation   Swisher et al. (2005) adapted from Kidder

Issue/ Problem	Dilemma	Distress	Temptation	Silence
Important values present	Two alternative courses of action: Right vs. Right decision	The right course of action is known but the clinician cannot perform it	Choice between right and wrong	Values are challenged but no one is speaking about this challenge to values

The Situation: _____

Rationale: _____

_____

_____

(continued on following page)

Ethical Principles and/or Standards of Ethical Conduct of the PTA (see Appendixes A and B)

Code of Ethics (Principles) for PTs	Rationale	Standards of Ethical Conduct (Standards) for PTAs	Rationale

Suggested Action:

CHAPTER 15

Professional Responsibility

All of us belong simultaneously to multiple communities. The most basic community is the one we are introduced to at birth, our family. It is the responsibility of the family unit to introduce a child to appropriate behavior and how to differentiate right from wrong. There are many other communities that a child will interact with on his or her way to adulthood—school, sports teams, band and chorus, religious groups, scouting—just to name a few. Entering a professional field is different, as the customary norms that apply to human interactions take on a higher level of obligation because of the very complex but most important patient–therapist relationship. All physical therapists are bound by the laws in the jurisdiction in which they practice and the Code of Ethics for the physical therapist. While both are binding the law is the minimum standard that must be adhered to, the Code of Ethics is more aspirational, but not optional, providing guidance on all aspects of the patient-therapist relationship. It is incumbent on students and licensed PTs and PTAs to know their state practice act, as well as the Code of Ethics. The public expects that we will demonstrate through our behavior the virtues of the profession as well as the Code of Ethics that incorporates the virtues of *accountability, altruism, compassion, excellence, integrity, professional duty, collaboration,* and *social responsibility.* Professional responsibility occurs in the individual, organization, and societal realms. The public may not understand excellence in the delivery of physical therapy, but they do recognize a breach of professional responsibility on the part of their physical therapy practitioner.

The cases presented here look at the importance of professional responsibility from several different perspectives.

Cases in this section:

A Passive Protocol   **Autonomous clinical decision making**

Artificial Competence   **Assessing competence and limitations**

Alphabet Soup   **Protect patients by accurate reporting of skills**

Moral Injury   **The importance of self-care**

Case Example 17

A PASSIVE PROTOCOL
Autonomous clinical decision making

It is the professional duty of physical therapists (PTs) to evaluate patients and clients and devise plans for their optimal plan of care by fully employing their knowledge, training, and skills. In some instances, however, their ability to do so may be blocked by those in positions of authority. Consider the following scenario.

Jill is a physical therapist who has practiced in the home care setting for the past five years. She loves the independence, variety, and challenges, so, when she decides to relocate upstate to live closer to her family, she applies exclusively to home healthcare agencies.

Her new employer is about the same size as her previous one, and Jill quickly feels accepted by her colleagues and clients. When it comes time for her first-month probation meeting, however, she senses that Bob, the physical therapy supervisor, isn't completely pleased with her work. When he says she's "by and large" doing a good job, she suppresses her surprise and disappointment—she had received nothing but praise from her previous employer—and asks what she might do to improve her performance.

Bob hesitates for a moment then says, "Don't get me wrong. Patients and staff like you. You're a talented PT. But we've been getting some heat from the physicians at the Orthopedic Group regarding your documentation when it comes to patients, they've referred to us after TKR [total knee replacement]."

Jill is perplexed. She takes pride in her documentation and makes certain that everything she does is meticulously recorded. "Heat?" she asks, repeating Bob's word. "Regarding what aspect of my documentation?"

"Specifically," Bob replies, "your documentation for two patients with TKR—Lucy Weber and Don Engels. In both cases, the Orthopedic Group's plan of care called for use of CPM [the continuous passive motion machine]. The group refers a lot of patients with TKRs to us," Bob notes, "and they believe that having PTs monitor use of CPM for thirty minutes of the session is key to the effective management of patients who are discharged from the hospital directly to home care. That belief is reflected in our agency's protocol for CPM use."

Jill breathes a slight sigh of relief, confident in her decisions and her ability to amply justify her actions. "Both Lucy and Don were only one week post-op when they came to us," Jill notes. "On my initial visit, I did make sure that both of them knew how to use the CPM, and at the end of each subsequent visit I've ensured that the machine is properly adjusted. "But," she continues, "there now is a body of research indicating that CPM offers no immediate functional recovery benefit in postoperative management of patients who've had an uncomplicated TKR. In fact, I just recently read an excellent research article on that subject in the *Journal of Arthroplasty*. The authors determined that, in fact, swelling persisted *longer* with CPM use. I also recently noticed that this very practice—use of CPM after uncomplicated TKR—is listed amount the 'Five Things Physical Therapists and Patients Should Question' by the APTA Center for Integrity in Practice. A phrase that sticks with me from that listing is that the 'limited benefits of CPM should be carefully weighed against the costs.'"

Bob responds, "I appreciate what you're saying, but you need also to weigh the fact that the Orthopedic Group is a strong proponent of CPM and doesn't take kindly to questioning of what it considers to be a proven protocol."

Jill is shocked that Bob doesn't appear to be supporting her actions, even after she's explained her reasoning and documentation. For her to spend thirty minutes of every forty-five-minute physical therapy session monitoring the work of a machine that offers questionable value—rather than spending that time using her knowledge and skills to get patients moving—seems to be against best practice—and thus against her patients' best interests. She elects, however, simply to acknowledge Bob's concerns, without challenging him.

On her next visit to the homes of Lucy and Don, she tells them that the physician group advocates CPM use and feels using the machine will benefit them. Jill also makes clear, however, that she firmly believes that CPM use should be limited, and that the interventions she is providing during her visits, combined with the extensive exercise program she has prescribed, offer the best opportunity for good results. She carefully explains her reasoning, citing both the research literature and the stance of her professional organization, APTA.

Two weeks go by. Then, once again, Bob calls Jill into her office. "Jim Baines from the Orthopedic Group called me up yesterday and was very upset that you're not following the protocol regarding CPM," he says. "He feels it's a disservice to patients. He also said that Lucy Weber called him, expressing confusion as to whether, or to what extent, she should be using the machine."

Jill cannot mask her frustration as she asks, "How does it make sense for me to passively watch a machine—one that, in fact, may be doing my patients more harm than good—rather than doing the job I'm trained to do?"

Bob looks directly at Jill, choosing his words carefully. "As I said when you and I met a couple of weeks ago, everyone likes you and you're doing good work. But the Orthopedic Group believes in this plan of care, and we've adopted their CPM protocol. Please understand that this isn't negotiable. We're part of a healthcare team, with physicians and others. And all of us at this practice would very much like for you to remain a member of our team. That's the bottom line, okay?"

Jill nods, but her head is spinning as she leaves Bob's office. How can she be true to her responsibilities and professional ethics as a PT while providing an intervention that is not well supported in the literature? Is her employer really prepared to fire her if she does not comply? Is she prepared to look for a new job if Bob continues to insist that she should follow this protocol rather than using her best professional judgment?

CONSIDER AND REFLECT

Jill consulted the evidence and the advice of her professional organization in taking the actions she took with her patients Lucy and Don. Jill is confident that the literature is on her side in the approach she has taken to Lucy's and Don's care. She has made her case to Bob, but he has not been swayed. A review of her ethical obligations as a PT should govern her next step.

After working through the ethical decision-making process, what course of action would you suggest?

Ethical Decision-Making Worksheet

Case: _____

The Realm   Jack Glaser (1994)

Individual	Organizational/ Institutional	Societal
The good of the patient/ client and focuses on rights, duties, relationships, and behaviors between individuals	Good of the organization, focuses on structures and systems, which facilitate organizational or institutional goals	Concerned with the common good

The Realm: _____

Rationale:

The Individual Process   James Rest (1994, 1999)

Moral Sensitivity	Moral Judgment	Moral Motivation	Moral Courage	Moral Potency (Hannah and Avolio, 2010)
Recognizing, interpreting, and framing an ethical situation	Right vs. wrong actions. Generating options, selecting and applying ethical principles	Priority on ethical values over other values. Professionalism is a primary motivator for ethical behavior	Implementing the chosen ethical action, development of a plan	Includes decision making that includes moral ownership, courage, and self-efficacy

(continued on following page)

The Individual Process: _____

Rationale:

The Situation   Swisher et al. (2005) adapted from Kidder

Issue/ Problem	Dilemma	Distress	Temptation	Silence
Important values present	Two alternative courses of action: Right vs. Right decision	The right course of action is known but the clinician cannot perform it	Choice between right and wrong	Values are challenged but no one is speaking about this challenge to values

The Situation: _____

Rationale:

Ethical Principles and/or Standards of Ethical Conduct of the PTA (see Appendixes A and B)

Code of Ethics (Principles) for PTs	Rationale	Standards of Ethical Conduct (Standards) for PTAs	Rationale

Suggested Action:

Case Example 18

ARTIFICIAL COMPETENCE
Assessing competence and limitations

Graduating from an accredited physical therapist (PT) education program and successfully completing the National Physical Therapy Exam suggest entry-level competence, and our skill set as PTs sharpens and expands with experience. Given physical therapy's broad scope of practice, however, is it reasonable to assume that PTs can be all things to all people who need our services?

Anita, a PT with eight years of experience, works at a PT-owned private practice that serves patients and clients of all ages who have orthopedic issues. Carl, the founder and owner, has built the practice into a trusted and valued community resource over the course of his twenty-year stewardship.

He has been telling staff for some time, however, that the practice needs to respond in a meaningful way to the economic challenges and opportunities presented by the Affordable Care Act and related changes in healthcare. "We must explore ways of expanding our patent and client base," he has said.

One Monday morning, Carl excitedly approaches Anita with some news. During the state chapter meeting that all the practice's PTs had attended over the weekend, Carl had met with Rita, a prosthetist who had exhibited. The upshot of their conversation is that the prosthetist will soon be referring some of her patients to the clinic.

Anita considers this development but does not share Carl's enthusiasm. She assumes that the reason Carl is telling her this news is that he knows she has treated some patients fitted with prosthetic limbs. But that was more than nine years ago, during her second clinical affiliation while she was still in school! Anita is aware, too, that none of her colleagues at the clinic have any experience with patients or clients who have prosthetic limbs.

"Do you think anyone here has the necessary background to work with such patients effectively?" Anita asks. "I mean, you know that my experience was limited and happened a long time ago, right?"

Carl smiles, pats her shoulder and says, "It's like riding a bicycle, Anita. When you see that patient in front of you, it'll all come back to you and you'll know what to do." She doesn't share Carl's confidence, but neither does she feel comfortable further challenging him. She'll catch up on the latest literature and research related to prosthetics and physical therapy, she reasons, and will defer further comment until the initial referral comes her way.

A few weeks go by without a patient from the prosthetist. Anita hopes the pledge was as ephemeral as a handshake. She has been doing a lot of reading, and she has discovered that prosthetic design—and even much of the terminology related to treatment of patients with prosthetic limbs—has changed markedly in the near-decade since she last worked with this patient population. She has a lot to learn, she realizes.

But then the day comes. Anita is assigned to work with Bill, who is 58 and recently has lost his right leg to complications from diabetes. He's friendly and has a positive attitude toward rehab, but his is not an easy case. Bill has circulatory insufficiency in his intact left leg and sensory loss in all four extremities. He's overweight. He has vision issues that affect his balance. Anita quickly sees that Bill isn't someone she can help leverage the counter near the sink in the examination room, then give a walker. He'll need considerably more stability before gait training with his prosthetic leg can safely begin.

The first thing she needs to do, Anita determines, is to call Rita, the prosthetist, for more information about Bill's artificial leg, as it is a model with which she is unfamiliar. Rita offers to hand-deliver the prosthetic to the clinic for Bill's next physical therapy session, so that she can instruct both Anita and Bill in its design and best use. Anita agrees, although she hopes Rita's presence won't in any way undermine Bill's confidence in Anita's ability to treat him.

Anita needn't have worried. Bill is happy to see two professionals working in tandem toward his optimal recovery. And Rita is very helpful, sharing everything the PT and patient need to know about safe use of the artificial limb. This information only amplifies Anita's concerns, however. For one thing, Bill first will need to stand with the new limb while supported by parallel equipment the clinic does not have. Also, Bill's optimal safety, Anita believes, dictates that she be by his side for the vast majority of the time he's at the clinic—a difficult proposition given the clinic's caseload. What it boils down to in Anita's mind is that her facility is not a good setting for this type of patient—in terms of clinical expertise, equipment, or logistics.

Later that day, Anita shares with Carl her concerns. He listens intently and without interruption. She is hopeful that she has swayed his thinking. But what he says next is, "We're physical therapists, Anita. We're professionals and problem solvers. I have every confidence in you. This clinic needs to establish new lines of referral, and I know we have the right team in place. This patient population is a great place to start."

Carl has made his position clear, and he's the boss. But Anita remains uneasy, unconvinced by the owner's assurances that everything will be fine.

CONSIDER AND REFLECT

Questioning her own competence to effectively treat Bill, Anita reaches out to Rita for help. That meeting does greatly clarify what Anita needs to do, and the resources she'll need in order to do it. That knowledge only heightens her concerns, however, as Carl does not share Anita's assessment that Bill's needs and the clinic's makeup are less than an ideal fit. While maintaining and developing revenue streams is important to the financial health of any physical therapy practice, the onus is on every PT to critically access and evaluate his or her personal scope of practice (skill and comfort level), and on every practice owner or director to make a similar assessment of the facility's staff expertise and logistic and material capabilities. Additional education and training of staff, as well as improvements in facility infrastructure, may be needed before safe and effective care can be provided.

After working through the ethical decision-making process, what course of action would you suggest?

Ethical Decision-Making Worksheet

Case: _____

The Realm   Jack Glaser (1994)

Individual	Organizational/Institutional	Societal
The good of the patient/ client and focuses on rights, duties, relationships, and behaviors between individuals	Good of the organization, focuses on structures and systems, which facilitate organizational or institutional goals	Concerned with the common good

The Realm: _____

Rationale:

The Individual Process   James Rest (1994, 1999)

Moral Sensitivity	Moral Judgment	Moral Motivation	Moral Courage	Moral Potency (Hannah and Avolio, 2010)
Recognizing, interpreting, and framing an ethical situation	Right vs. wrong actions. Generating options, selecting and applying ethical principles	Priority on ethical values over other values. Professionalism is a primary motivator for ethical behavior	Implementing the chosen ethical action, development of a plan	Includes decision making that includes moral ownership, courage, and self-efficacy

(continued on following page)

The Individual Process: _____

Rationale:

The Situation

Swisher et al. (2005) adapted from Kidder

Issue/ Problem	Dilemma	Distress	Temptation	Silence
Important values present	Two alternative courses of action: Right vs. Right decision	The right course of action is known but the clinician cannot perform it	Choice between right and wrong	Values are challenged but no one is speaking about this challenge to values

The Situation: _____

Rationale:

Ethical Principles and/or Standards of Ethical Conduct of the PTA (see Appendixes A and B)

Code of Ethics (Principles) for PTs	Rationale	Standards of Ethical Conduct (Standards) for PTAs	Rationale

Suggested Action:

Case Example 19

ALPHABET SOUP
Protect patients by accurate reporting of skills

The best physical therapists (PTs) and physical therapist assistants (PTAs) never stop learning. But what's the best way to convey such dedication to the public? Consider the following scenario.

David directs and is a staff PT at the Jonesville clinic of Excellent Physical Therapy, a PT-owned network of twelve facilities in three adjoining states. He's occasionally ribbed about the business's name, which some people find hyperbolic or pretentious, but David is genuinely proud of the care provided and the professionalism displayed by staff at his site and the other Excellent branches he's visited over the years. His typical response to all good-natured jibes is, "When we say 'Excellent', it's not just a name. It's a promise."

David takes particular pride in his staff's dedication to continuing education, which reflects their drive to enhance their knowledge and skills. He is one of five PTs at the Jonesville site, all of whom are supported by a PTA. The staff annually exhausts the clinic's continuing education (CE) budget, and everyone takes additional courses at their own expense. One of the PTs graduated school as a Doctor of Physical Therapy, a second PT earned a transitional DPT while employed at the Jonesville clinic, a third is certified orthopedic clinical specialist, and both David and the remaining PT have more than ten years of experience in the profession. The PTA is certified in lymphedema management and has earned PTA Recognition of Advanced Proficiency from APTA in three different areas of physical therapy. Pointing to these facts, David sometimes observes, "We don't use the word 'excellent' lightly around here."

Staff from all of the clinics meet two weekends a year at one of the clinic sites for a combination business meeting, brainstorming session, and daylong CE course. David always finds these gatherings to be great opportunities to bond with colleagues, get the latest company news, and, most importantly, learn new things through the coursework and through the exchange of ideas. So, he's energized when he drives to a neighboring state for the latest event. This time the CE course, taught by a senior partner of the company, is titled MOVE—for Movement Options and Victory through Exercise.

David completes the course-concluding exam and claims his certificate. He always finds something beneficial in a CE course, even when it doesn't tell him that much that's completely new to him. It may offer him a slightly different way of looking at a familiar issue, or prompt a comment from a colleague that piques his interest and, perhaps, further research. Every CE course a PT or PTA can take is helpful in some way, David believes—even though he and other staff sometimes joke that they could wallpaper the clinic with their cumulative stack of CE certificates.

The next day, however, things take an odd and unexpected turn. The company's owner, Paul, gets up during the business meeting and announces a number of changes that the management team has drafted. They are designed to counter what Paul says is a troubling trend in public perception. The company's analytic data indicate that Excellent Physical Therapy has seen a slight downturn in market share that may be attributable to public perception that other facilities have better-qualified staff. A number of area physical therapy practices, chiropractic clinics, and high-end gyms seem to be attracting consumers by highlighting in their advertising such words as "experience" and "training." A "counteroffensive" is needed, Paul says.

"Listen," the owner prefaces his remarks, "we're all justifiably proud of the work we do and the quality and value we offer. The steps the management team is advocating in no way are meant to be seen as any comment on the amazing job that you do." David and his colleagues shoot each other quizzical glances, as if to ask, "Where's he going with this?" The answer quickly follows.

Henceforth, Paul announces, all corporate advertising will refer to Excellent Physical Therapy's PTs as "doctors" and "specialists." CE certificates will be prominently displayed at all sites, and all PTs and PTAs will be expected to add to their business cards and website biographies all of their CE-conferred credentials, such as this weekend's "MOVE" designation for having successfully completed the course.

When a PT jokes half-seriously that "some of us will have *War and Peace* after our names now," Paul responds, "I think a lot of people find those letters reassuring, even if they don't really know what they mean."

"Not that I exactly want to call this to your attention, Paul, but not all of us here are doctors," another PT points out, to a smattering of nervous laughter.

"You've got nothing to worry about!" Paul parries with a smile. "The fact is, about 60% of our therapists are DPTs, and every single PT we have on staff, regardless of degree status, is a highly skilled professional. Yes, it's true that some of us attended school in a different era and haven't yet had the opportunity to go back for our transitional degree. Guilty as charged!" he concedes with a laugh. "But, look. All of us practice at a very high level. That's what we need to convey to the public. We're all specialists in one way or another, and we're all the products of our continuing education."

Back at the Jonesville clinic early Monday morning, David stands before his staff to discuss what transpired over the weekend. Some people have already shared their concerns with him privately. He starts by saying, "I hear your reservations about the marketing direction that Paul outlined to me, it smacks of misrepresentation. It strikes me as unethical and perhaps illegal. Now, with all of that said, I'm open to suggestions as to what we might do about it. I'm sure everyone in this room agrees that we provide excellent physical therapy. But if we fight this, we just might run the risk of becoming excellent out-of-work PTs and PTAs. So, I'm opening the floor for discussion."

CONSIDER AND REFLECT

Both the Code of Ethics for the Physical Therapist and the Standards of Ethical Conduct for the Physical Therapist Assistant direct practitioners to "demonstrate integrity" in their relationships with patients, clients, and the public. It is important to note, as well, that many states limit identifying letters to the regulatory designator (PT or PTA) and the highest educational degree achieved, and some states require that additional identifiers be fully explained, to ensure that consumers understand their meaning.

What if the marketing "pitch," agreed upon by the Excellent Physical Therapy management team were to be, "Our network's PTs have a doctorate?" Similarly, who is to say what constitutes being a "specialist," or which professional credentials are the most meaningful to consumers? On the other hand, are the management team's mandates ethically compatible with APTA core documents? Might the practice acts in the three relevant states have legal bearing on this public relations initiative?

After working through the ethical decision-making process, what course of action would you suggest?

Ethical Decision-Making Worksheet

Case: _____

The Realm   Jack Glaser (1994)

Individual	Organizational/ Institutional	Societal
The good of the patient/ client and focuses on rights, duties, relationships, and behaviors between individuals	Good of the organization, focuses on structures and systems, which facilitate organizational or institutional goals	Concerned with the common good

The Realm: _____

Rationale:

The Individual Process   James Rest (1994, 1999)

Moral Sensitivity	Moral Judgment	Moral Motivation	Moral Courage	Moral Potency (Hannah and Avolio, 2010)
Recognizing, interpreting, and framing an ethical situation	Right vs. wrong actions. Generating options, selecting and applying ethical principles	Priority on ethical values over other values. Professionalism is a primary motivator for ethical behavior	Implementing the chosen ethical action, development of a plan	Includes decision making that includes moral ownership, courage, and self-efficacy

(continued on following page)

The Individual Process: _____

Rationale:

The Situation   Swisher et al. (2005) adapted from Kidder

Issue/ Problem	Dilemma	Distress	Temptation	Silence
Important values present	Two alternative courses of action: Right vs. Right decision	The right course of action is known but the clinician cannot perform it	Choice between right and wrong	Values are challenged but no one is speaking about this challenge to values

The Situation: _____

Rationale:

Ethical Principles and/or Standards of Ethical Conduct of the PTA (see Appendixes A and B)

Code of Ethics (Principles) for PTs	Rationale	Standards of Ethical Conduct (Standards) for PTAs	Rationale

Suggested Action:

Case Example 20

MORAL INJURY
The importance of self-care

The impact of the pandemic, payment issues, productivity demands, and an unsettled health care environment have generated considerable discussion about clinician burnout over the past few years. The concept of moral injury has been introduced into this dialogue, speaking to the condition that affects the provider's ability to provide their expected high-quality care, resulting in a conflict between what is required of the clinician and their "calling" to help people. While moral injury certainly has a profound impact on the individual PT or PTA, there are related consequences on patients and colleagues that impact the safe, effective, and ethical delivery of care.

Larry, a PT, and Dave, a PTA, have worked together at Tall Pines Restorative Care for almost seven years. The two men are close in age and share not only a love for their chosen profession, but a passion for golf and all things football. They have seen their share of administrative changes, corporate buyouts, and shifting missions and directions, but with their focus on providing the best care possible for their patients, they took each change in stride. Looking back on the two years of uncertainty that COVID-19 caused in the industry, they felt pride in the care they provided while maintaining their personal safety and the safety of their families. During that time, they felt valued by the facility's administration and worked collaboratively with the rest of the health care team to provide for the patients at Tall Pines. They were not particularly worried when they were informed at the beginning of the year that Tall Pines had decided to contract its rehabilitation services—physical therapy, occupational therapy, and speech language pathology—to an outside agency. They were assured that the terms of the contract outlined that they were to be offered a position with the contract agency at the same salary. Larry and Dave were a team, and they were confident that this change was one, like so many others in their careers, that they could easily adapt to. The director of rehab, Melissa, herself a PT, decided this was a good time for her to make the move to a facility closer to home. They were assured by Sue, the regional manager of the contract company, that an experienced director would soon be appointed to manage rehab services, and the regional manager would take care of the day-to-day operations until that took place. While she was very pleasant, it was obvious that the regional manager knew little about subacute facilities and, unfortunately, even less about effective management. The previous director had carried three-quarters of a full caseload, which quickly became divided between Larry and Dave. Added to that, more patients were added to the caseload as COVID-19 fears abated, and demand for services increased. Banking on the goodwill of their longtime relationship with the facility administration, Larry and Dave went together to speak with the administrator to share their concerns about the decline in patient care they were already seeing: group therapy sessions with patients inappropriately paired, and little time for documentation, meeting patients' individual needs, following up on equipment, discharge planning, and the myriad other tasks associated with safe and effective care. The administrator's response made it clear that these decisions were now in the purview of the contract agency. Disheartened, Larry and Dave approached their colleagues in occupational therapy and speech language pathology and found they were equally alarmed at the lack of concern for patient care exhibited by their new employer. They knew that they were capable of providing much better care than they were currently giving, and they were determined to help their new managers see what could be done. As a team, they approached the regional manager, who listened but made it clear that these changes were necessary and consistent with industry standards, and they could either adapt or consider leaving. Larry and Dave decided that they have weathered changes before, and they would continue to do so with the focus on patient care guiding their decisions and judgment. The two colleagues often pointed to their guiding virtue of integrity, with the emphasis on the "grit" imbedded within the word.

Even after a new director of rehab was hired, conditions did not improve; there was no additional help in physical therapy as patient care demands continued to increase. Larry, as the evaluating PT, frequently found that his requests for time off were denied because there was no coverage. He had little time to do his own paperwork, let alone the review and signoff of Dave's documentation. Dave's frequent requests to "grab a round of golf after work" were turned down, with Larry citing he was "just too tired" or had "too much to do." He also was opting out of the weekly Monday Night Football viewing sessions they both usually looked forward to every season. Dave was concerned, not just about the social interaction that he was missing, but also about the decline in patient care that he was noticing and the impact it was having on his ability to do what was both expected and required of him as a PTA. Larry always had gone the extra mile for patients, but now he seemed willing to settle for less-than-optimal patient care. He rarely checked in on patients that he handed off to Dave, and the handoff of a new patient was nothing more than a perfunctory, "Read my initial evaluation; I don't have time to go over the details. You know what to do." While Dave appreciated the vote of confidence from his colleague, he did not appreciate the rationale for it. When Larry called out sick twice in one week and did not, despite reminders, sign off on Dave's notes for days or see all of his assigned patients, Dave became alarmed. His colleague, and his friend, was no longer performing as a competent PT.

Dave felt obligated to act. Dave approached Larry one morning about Larry's willingness to accept less than the excellence that the two had always held as a key value, and maybe even a loss of some of the grit that they found to be so important in maintaining their integrity. Larry did not disagree. He acknowledged his lack of interest, his fatigue, and even that he might be depressed—all classic signs of burnout. He also recognized that his actions had a profound impact on Dave's ability to do his job. From what Larry knew of burnout, it was best remedied by changing what you were doing. But as he considered his options, he knew he still very much wanted to be a PT. However, he didn't believe he could perform his job responsibilities at the standard he personally demanded of himself. He could not provide patient care or appropriately work with Dave under the conditions imposed on them. If this wasn't burnout, could it be moral injury? And how could Larry influence the situation so he could be the kind of physical therapist that he expected of himself while continuing to practice safely, effectively, and ethically?

CONSIDER AND REFLECT

Both Larry and Dave must make decisions that impact patient care. First, they each must consider their own relationship with the organization and the ability to make independent decisions in the patient's best interest. They also must consider their professional relationship and how their individual mental health may impact their colleagues and their patients. The situation raises issues of professional responsibility to themselves, colleagues, patients and the organization.

After working through the ethical decision-making process, what course of action would you suggest?

Ethical Decision-Making Worksheet

Case: _____

The Realm   Jack Glaser (1994)

Individual	Organizational/ Institutional	Societal
The good of the patient/ client and focuses on rights, duties, relationships and behaviors between individuals	Good of the organization, focuses on structures and systems, which facilitate organizational or institutional goals	Concerned with the common good

(continued on following page)

The Realm _____

Rationale:

The Individual Process: James Rest (1994, 1999)

Moral Sensitivity	Moral Judgment	Moral Motivation	Moral Courage	Moral Potency (Hannah and Avolio, 2010)
Recognizing, interpreting, and framing an ethical situation	Right versus wrong actions. Generating options, selecting and applying ethical principles	Priority on ethical values over other values. Professionalism is a primary motivator for ethical behavior	Implementing the chosen ethical action, development of a plan	Includes decision making that includes moral ownership, courage, and self-efficacy

The Individual Process: _____

Rationale:

The Situation: Swisher et al. (2005) adapted from Kidder

Issue/ Problem	Dilemma	Distress	Temptation	Silence
Important values present	Two alternative courses of action: Right vs. Right decision	The right course of action is known but the clinician cannot perform it	Choice between right and wrong	Values are challenged but no one is speaking about this challenge to values

The Situation: _____

Rationale:

_____

_____

_____

Ethical Principles and/or Standards of Ethical Conduct of the PTA (see Appendixes A and B)

(continued on following page)

Code of Ethics (Principles) for PTs	Rationale	Standards of Ethical Conduct (Standards) for PTAs	Rationale

Suggested Action:

CHAPTER 16

Professional Self-Regulation

Professionals are granted the privilege of monitoring themselves. This is in exchange for the safe and effective administering of the duties and responsibilities that are inherent in the care of patients. Self-monitoring is not just the responsibility of the regulatory authority; it is a duty every licensee has. Most physical therapy practice acts have within them a "duty to report." Our code of ethics also addresses this requirement to self-regulate stating that in Principles 5D and 5E, there is the requirement to provide assistance and, if necessary, contact authorities. So why is this particular responsibility so difficult for licensees to actually "do"? As a close-knit professional community, it is hard to report a colleague. Many of us are raised "not to tattle," but the stakes in those childhood encounters are significantly less than the stakes we now encounter with the central focus on the well-being of the patient. Reporting is not restricted to one way in which to report. The act that is of concern must be evaluated to determine the root cause so those observing the behaviors can determine the best way to address the problem. A physical therapist (PT) or physical therapist assistant (PTA) with substandard skills raises different concerns than the clinician who has a substance abuse problem or some cognition issues. There are several reasons why self-regulation is so important. The origin of the concept is based on trust. We say to the public through our principle-based ethical actions, we demonstrate respect for the patient (autonomy) we promise to use our knowledge and skills to do good for the patient (beneficence). We further promise not to harm a patient, (non-maleficence) and we ensure patients that we are honest (veracity) and will treat all entrusted to our care fairly (justice). This relationship is built and sustained on trust. The trust given to us to "keep our own house in order" is what we have to keep in mind when confronted with practitioners who have negated this trust in some way.

Each of the cases presented in this section speaks in a different way regarding the duty to report requirement.

Cases in this section:

Who Are You?	**Responsibility to report**
Where Is the Evidence?	**Exceeding responsibility**
An Education on Staff Behavior	**Stopping poor practice**
Independent or set adrift?	**Responsibility to know your practice requirements.**

Case Example 21

WHO ARE YOU?
Responsibility to report

A physical therapist (PT) develops a personal relationship not just with the patient but with the family. This relationship is built on trust. When there is a minor or adult who is not competently involved, this relationship becomes more complicated.

Sarah is a PT. She works in an outpatient pediatric clinic and loves the opportunities she has to really get to know her patients and their families. Her caseload includes the children she sees at home through early intervention as well as preschoolers all the way up to the few on program that are in middle school. She can't really decide which age she likes best, but she has learned to expect the unexpected regardless of which child she is with. One of the children who offered the biggest challenge to her was an eight-year-old boy Mikey who was very shy and never said a word for at least the first month she treated him. He recently moved from a nearby town and seemed to be very pensive. He was driven to therapy by his grandmother. Mikey cooperated but did the absolute minimum with very little interest and no carryover at home. Sarah was aware that his mother was away, but she wasn't privy to the circumstances surrounding her absence. She tried everything to get Mikey engaged, but he was obviously very unhappy. Suddenly one afternoon Mikey came bounding into the office. He looked like a different kid, and when Sarah went out to say hi to his grandmother, she was greeted by a younger version of his grandmother, obviously his mother. Mikey couldn't wait to show his mom what he was doing and was happy to participate in any activity Sarah asked him to do. At the end of the session Sarah welcomed her home, but Mikey's mom seemed to be very private, sharing nothing about her whereabouts. Mikey didn't seem to know very much either; he was just happy to have her home and he was like a changed child. Mikey became her most enthusiastic patient, willing to try new things and making progress. Mikey even seemed to be making some friends at school. Sarah wasn't ready to grapple with the decisions she was faced with after she was confronted with some information on her favorite TV show called Crime Abatement. The show broadcasts regional events and engages the community to assist law enforcement with identifying individuals that have warrants or other legal action against them that the police are unable to locate. Imagine Sarah's shock when she saw Mikey's mom on the show. She had a different last name than Mikey, but it was unmistakable; it was most definitely her and she was last seen in the town that Mikey had moved from. Her immediate thought was why hadn't she skipped the show this evening, ... could she pretend that she skipped the show and never saw the broadcast? Now that she was aware, did she have an obligation to report what she knows? She found it difficult to sleep that night and even harder to concentrate when she tried to work with Mikey the next day. She pondered, wasn't her first responsibility to her patient, she couldn't divulge information about him, it would be a HIPAA violation. She could certainly rationalize not reporting the information she knows to law enforcement because of the impact on the child, and he is her first, and only responsibility. While she could convince herself of the soundness of that argument, she could not help but think there is more to this, and while Mikey's well-being is of great importance is it her only responsibility as a citizen and as a PT?

CONSIDER AND REFLECT

Sarah determined that her primary responsibility is to her patient, but she had to decide if she could continue to fulfill that obligation and her civic responsibility as well. She realized that she did not have to divulge any PHI while reporting the whereabouts of the mother and she could ask for law enforcement not to come to the office so she could protect Mikey from having to witness his mother being taking into custody. That realization did not resolve all of the issues that she had concerns about, but it did provide her with a clearer focus. This is a complex situation involving trust between the PT, the patient, and the family as well as the integrity of the physical therapist as a member of the community. Sarah did not know the extent of the legal charges against the mother, but she was sure it wasn't a few parking ticket violations to make it to the Crime Abatement Program. As a citizen she knows her responsibility and as a PT she knows her responsibility. What she is unsure about is how to reconcile what she feels are conflicting obligations.

After working through the ethical decision-making process, what course of action would you suggest?

Ethical Decision-Making Worksheet

Case: _____

The Realm   Jack Glaser (1994)

Individual	Organizational/ Institutional	Societal
The good of the patient/ client and focuses on rights, duties, relationships, and behaviors between individuals	Good of the organization, focuses on structures and systems, which facilitate organizational or institutional goals	Concerned with the common good

(continued on following page)

The Realm: _____

Rationale:

The Individual Process   James Rest (1994, 1999)

Moral Sensitivity	Moral Judgment	Moral Motivation	Moral Courage	Moral Potency (Hannah and Avolio, 2010)
Recognizing, interpreting, and framing an ethical situation	Right vs. wrong actions. Generating options, selecting and applying ethical principles	Priority on ethical values over other values. Professionalism is a primary motivator for ethical behavior	Implementing the chosen ethical action, development of a plan	Includes decision making that includes moral ownership, courage, and self-efficacy

The Individual Process: _____

Rationale:

The Situation   Swisher et al. (2005) adapted from Kidder

Issue/ Problem	Dilemma	Distress	Temptation	Silence
Important values present	Two alternative courses of action: Right vs. Right decision	The right course of action is known but the clinician cannot perform it	Choice between right and wrong	Values are challenged but no one is speaking about this challenge to values

The Situation: _____

Rationale:

Ethical Principles and/or Standards of Ethical Conduct of the PTA (see Appendixes A and B)

Code of Ethics (Principles) for PTs	Rationale	Standards of Ethical Conduct (Standards) for PTAs	Rationale

(continued on following page)

Code of Ethics (Principles) for PTs	Rationale	Standards of Ethical Conduct (Standards) for PTAs	Rationale

Suggested Action:

Case Example 22

WHERE IS THE EVIDENCE?
Exceeding responsibility

What does "professional responsibility" ethically entail? It's a broad term that encompasses all aspects of professional behavior and the obligation to ensure that every patient and client receives safe and effective care. Consider the following scenario.

Lance, a physical therapist (PT) with a total of eight years' experience in a variety of practice settings, feels that he's secured his dream job when he's named director of physical therapy services at the Brunswick Comprehensive Care Community.

The one-time nursing home has been extensively remodeled and modernized in recent years under new ownership. It offers residents an array of living arrangements—independent and assisted living, nursing, and memory care—under a common roof. Lance leads a staff of seven PTs and three physical therapist assistants (PTAs), a few of whom have been employed at Brunswick since its creation in 1985. Facilities include a six-bed subacute unit, an outpatient clinic, a thirty-bed skilled nursing unit, and a 10-bed memory care wing.

Lance's predecessor, Ray, had left under murky circumstances. He'd been cordial and helpful to Lance during the transition and had told Lance that his family was relocating to live nearer to his aging in-laws. But Lance sensed from management that Ray, who'd been at Brunswick since 1998, had been slow to adapt to the expansion of services and was uneasy about plans to break ground on a new building adjacent to the existing one. Lance believes that the parting of ways was at best a mutual decision, but that Ray probably was forced out.

Lance has been mentored at each of his previous jobs by forward-looking PTs, has taken a multitude of professional development courses on the latest developments in geriatrics and practice management, and has given stockpiling ideas for a comprehensive professional development program that he plans to implement at Brunswick.

After spending his first month on the job getting to know staff, residents, and the facility itself, Lance is ready to share his plans. During the Monday-morning staff meeting, he delivers an impassioned speech about the importance of up-to-the-minute, evidence-based practice. Lance lays out plans for a weekly "journal club" in which staff will take turns talking about pertinent research, and a monthly in-service during which staff will share what they've learned in recent professional development courses. "We'll all learn together, and our residents will reap the benefits!" he exclaims.

While a few staff are visibly excited by these plans, overall the initial reaction is muted. Lance isn't discouraged, however. He knows that continuing education requirements are fairly minimal in their state, that his predecessor had not emphasized coursework, and that staff aren't used to commanding the floor and talking about research and developments within the profession.

Lance asks individual staff members to sign up for weekly journal club leadership, and to indicate which courses interest them from an array listed on a handout. This exercise opens up discussion, with some people volunteering that "I've really been wanting to get up to speed on this subject," and others recalling, "I read something about this study that I think would be perfect for our discussion." Before long, everyone has chimed into—and seemingly brought into—Lance's education program.

Everyone, that is, except Sid, a PT who remains silent and looks frankly bored by the discussion. Lance decides to let it pass as Sid is one of the original Brunswick staffers and undoubtedly is a bit set in his ways. As Lance's program unfolds and an environment of collective learning is fostered, Sid likely will get into the spirit, Lance reasons.

But in the following month, such optimism is not borne out. In fact, not only does Sid remain detached during journal club and the in-service meeting, but also his behavior causes Lance to look into and uncover some troubling aspects of Sid's work. He consistently has the highest number of no-show and cancelled appointments among staff, according to records, and, even more disturbing, he has a pattern of delivering more or less the same interventions, regardless of circumstances, and of insufficiently progressing his patients.

Lance asks Tammy—who, like Sid, had been one of Brunswick's very first PTs—for her assessment of her coworker's care provision and attitude. "All I'll say," she responds, "is that my philosophy is to never stop learning, while Sid's is 'Never stop doing what you've always been doing.' Which, I have to say, tends to be as little as possible."

Lance is taken aback by Tammy's words. He's not sure what upsets him more—Sid's pattern of substandard patient care and lack of interest in growing professionally, or the suggestion that Sid's behaviors are widely acknowledged and tolerated by his coworkers. Clearly, Lance sees, it is his responsibility as director of physical therapy to address these issues.

CONSIDER AND REFLECT

Lance has correctly concluded that doing nothing is not an option. He could simply fire Sid. Or, if Sid is amenable to remediation, Lance could see that Sid gets the instruction and guidance he needs to change his behaviors and mindset in ways that ensure safe and effective care—with the understanding that failure to reform will mean termination. Lance also could articulate a zero-tolerance policy toward substandard performance and institute guidelines for confidential reporting.

Lance knew he would face challenges in his new job, but with committed ownership and a veteran staff, he hadn't anticipated such an immediate and disturbing leadership test.

After working through the ethical decision-making process, what course of action would you suggest?

Ethical Decision-Making Worksheet

Case: _____

The Realm   Jack Glaser (1994)

Individual	Organizational/ Institutional	Societal
The good of the patient/client and focuses on rights, duties, relationships, and behaviors between individuals	Good of the organization, focuses on structures and systems, which facilitate organizational or institutional goals	Concerned with the common good

The Realm: _____

Rationale:

The Individual Process   James Rest (1994, 1999)

(continued on following page)

Moral Sensitivity	Moral Judgment	Moral Motivation	Moral Courage	Moral Potency (Hannah and Avolio, 2010)
Recognizing, interpreting, and framing an ethical situation	Right vs. wrong actions. Generating options, selecting and applying ethical principles	Priority on ethical values over other values. Professionalism is a primary motivator for ethical behavior	Implementing the chosen ethical action, development of a plan	Includes decision making that includes moral ownership, courage, and self-efficacy

The Individual Process: _____

Rationale:

The Situation   Swisher et al. (2005) adapted from Kidder

Issue/ Problem	Dilemma	Distress	Temptation	Silence
Important values present	Two alternative courses of action: Right vs. Right decision	The right course of action is known but the clinician cannot perform it	Choice between right and wrong	Values are challenged but no one is speaking about this challenge to values

The Situation: _____

Rationale:

Ethical Principles and/or Standards of Ethical Conduct of the PTA (see Appendixes A and B)

Code of Ethics (Principles) for PTs	Rationale	Standards of Ethical Conduct (Standards) for PTAs	Rationale

(continued on following page)

Suggested Action:

Case Example 23

AN EDUCATION ON STAFF BEHAVIOR
Stopping poor practice

Failure to act on warning signs related to an employee's behavior not only is unwise but is also unethical, and it may have profound societal repercussions. Consider the following scenario.

Sarah is a longtime supervisor at Prime Time Therapy Services in upstate New York. Carol is in her third week at the practice. Late one morning, Carol steps into Sarah's office, holding a newspaper. She closes the door behind her and asks if Sarah has read or heard about the arrest of a physical therapist (PT) who has been charged with molesting a thirteen-year-old patient in the outpatient department of a local hospital.

"I can't imagine anyone in our profession violating the public's trust in such a horrible way," says visibly shaken Carol.

"Unfortunately, there are predators in all walks of life," Sarah responds. "But you're right—if it's true, it's shocking."

Carol, a new graduate who recently earned her Doctor of Physical Therapy degree from a university in California and moved East to join her fiancé, asks, "I'm curious, since you've been a PT in this area for a long time have you ever run into this PT?" She reads from the newspaper a name Sarah doesn't recognize. There is no photo of the accused PT in the article.

"No, it doesn't ring a bell," Sarah answers.

A few hours later, however, something kicks in, and she realizes that not only has she crossed paths with the man she knew by an abbreviation of the middle name cited in the newspaper article, but that he actually worked at Prime Time briefly about five years ago. She can picture him in her head but can't immediately recall much about him or his tenure at the practice. At the end of the day, she seeks out Tim, a veteran physical therapist at Prime Time with whom she sometimes reminisces about "the old days."

Tim is surprised that Sarah's memory of their one-time colleague seems fuzzy. "Don't you remember that time I told you I overheard him seeming to be coming on to a patient who couldn't have been more than 12?" he asks. "The guy denied it, of course, and said I'd misheard him and taken things out of context. I also told you about the time I suspected he'd taken a photo of a young girl while she was doing her exercises on a mat, because when I came into the room, he stuffed his phone into his pocket and looked all nervous."

"Oh my gosh, yes!" Sarah now recalls. "You know, I'd talked to him about those incidents, and I wasn't completely satisfied with his answers. I'd never seen any suspect behavior myself, but you weren't the only person working here back then who shared suspicions with me. He was a smooth talker, but I was thinking of putting him on probation when he told me he was leaving after only having been here for, what, four months? I just kind of thought, 'Good riddance.'"

"In fact, when another clinic called me for a reference," she now recalls, "I certainly wasn't effusive, but I was factual about what I saw as being his strengths. I felt uncomfortable mentioning the other stuff because it was unproven. I don't know if he ultimately got that job, but obviously he found his way to the hospital at some point.

There's an uncomfortable silence as both Tim and Sarah simultaneously wonder if Sarah might somehow have altered the course of subsequent events. "What could I have done differently?" she asks herself, feeling guilty about her inaction. "What if I'd really tried to get to the bottom of people's suspicions? What if that had led to my firing the guy? What effect might that have had? Should I have reported him to law enforcement, even though all I had was 'smoke' but no 'fire'? What were my ethical obligations in that situation?"

Tim starts putting on his coat to go home. "Well, you never really know about people, or what they might do," he says uneasily, in a way that tells Sarah he neither is absolving nor completely indicting her.

"No, I suppose you don't," she responds.

CONSIDER AND REFLECT

The therapist had been charged with child molestation. He had at least three employers, and perhaps more. If other supervisors had been made aware of issues similar to those that were reported to Sarah, but if they, like her, took definitive action now, might such collective passivity have a profound effect on patient care? Poor practitioners exist in every profession; there are safeguards in place to protect the public, such as reporting well-founded suspicions and being honest and truthful when asked about an employee that you have concerns about. Passing on a problem to another agency spreads a wider net of inappropriate behavior.

After working through the ethical decision-making process, what course of action would you suggest?

Ethical Decision-Making Worksheet

Case: _____

The Realm   Jack Glaser (1994)

(continued on following page)

Individual	Organizational/ Institutional	Societal
The good of the patient/ client and focuses on rights, duties, relationships, and behaviors between individuals	Good of the organization, focuses on structures and systems, which facilitate organizational or institutional goals	Concerned with the common good

The Realm: _____

Rationale:

The Individual Process: James Rest (1994, 1999)

Moral Sensitivity	Moral Judgment	Moral Motivation	Moral Courage	Moral Potency (Hannah and Avolio, 2010)
Recognizing, interpreting, and framing an ethical situation	Right vs. wrong actions. Generating options, selecting and applying ethical principles	Priority on ethical values over other values. Professionalism is a primary motivator for ethical behavior	Implementing the chosen ethical action, development of a plan	Includes decision making that includes moral ownership, courage, and self-efficacy

The Individual Process: _____

Rationale:

The Situation   Swisher et al. (2005) adapted from Kidder

Issue/ Problem	Dilemma	Distress	Temptation	Silence
Important values present	Two alternative courses of action: Right vs. Right decision	The right course of action is known but the clinician cannot perform it	Choice between right and wrong	Values are challenged but no one is speaking about this challenge to values

The Situation: _____

Rationale:

Ethical Principles and/or Standards of Ethical Conduct of the PTA (see Appendixes A and B)

(continued on following page)

Code of Ethics (Principles) for PTs	Rationale	Standards of Ethical Conduct (Standards) for PTAs	Rationale

Suggested Action:

Case Example 24

INDEPENDENT OR SET ADRIFT?
Responsibility to know your practice act

Scott was one of those PT students that knew before he started school that he wanted to work in pediatrics and though it was not where he started his career, he was very grateful for the experience that he had in both subacute and outpatient for the five years before he decided to take the plunge and pursue his dream of working in a school setting with children. He considered himself very fortunate because the large hospital system that he worked in had a pediatric rehab facility and he rotated through the unit several times reinforcing his pediatric skills but more important than that, solidifying his desire to eventually devote himself full time to the pediatric population. He geared his continuing competence activities between improving his abilities in his current work environment and planning for his future pediatric career. He already started investigating what the requirements would be to get his Pediatric Clinical Specialist certification. The recent disruptions in clinical practice that arose from the COVID pandemic put his active pursuit of a school-based position on hold but as things sometimes happen a school position seemed to drop in his lap late in the Spring, and after a short discussion with his fiancé he decided it was now or never making the change for the new school year starting in August. While he would be the only PT in the two schools he was assigned to, he easily connected with the other PTs in the district and found them more than helpful with tips on the best equipment to outfit himself with and how to navigate the many nuances of the new school year. Scott was accustomed to having a designated treatment area, and even when he treated bedside he had a home base in the building, the PT gym, but he found the school to be a maze of areas that he was welcome to use … if nobody else was in there at that time, a caveat that required a lot of flexibility on his part in a busy school environment. His colleagues advised him to stake a claim early in the year to the multipurpose room, or the gym during lunch periods, or the lunchroom during class times, and if all else fails find a nice quiet stairwell with little traffic that he could call his own. Scott immediately embraced the creativity and adaptability that was demanded by his new setting and realized that he was expected to be very independent in his practice. The first two weeks before school started Scott was busy reading the Individualized Education Plans (IEP) or 504 Plans for each of his students, and in negotiating for scheduled times to pull his students out of class or plan to work with them in the classroom setting as dictated by their written plans. Scott was no stranger to the importance of a structured care plan, he was quite adept at using the electronic medical record system at the hospital, but navigating the complexities of these plans was initially a bit daunting. He contacted Gloria one of the PTs in the district who encouraged him to call if he had any questions and she was good to her word, trying to help him nego-tiate the nuances of the school setting. The PTs in the district were working for an agency called Kids Plus, based in another state but contracting PTs and OT's into school districts and early intervention. Though Scott was excited about the professional independence of the school setting, he was very grateful for Gloria's willingness to provide some counsel. With Gloria's help Scott realized that the IEP and the 504 plan contained the guidelines he had to use to develop his treatment schedule, two individual sessions per week for 30 minutes vs. one individual and one group session. This called for a spread sheet and Scott dug into the challenge of making sure he complied with the requirements dictated by the district's legal agreement for services the children were promised to receive. While his schedule looked good on paper as Scott began seeing the children some of the plans did not seem to make a lot of good treatment sense. Based on his early assessment, some of the children needed more than the plan called for and some needed far less or a different type of intervention, in class or pull out. His call to Gloria confirmed for him that sometimes the plan was a bit outdated, kids changed quickly and particularly during this past year where much of the instruction had been remote. Not knowing the children, Gloria suggested that he speak with his colleagues in the building in OT and Speech and the Child Study Team (CST) to see what their thoughts were about some of the children he was having difficulty rationalizing the prescribed plan with the child's needs. Her closing remark, "just remember you are no longer in the medical model as a PT, you are an ancillary service," resonated with Scott as he tried to reconcile what he was finding with what he was obligated to do. Scott was well aware that PT and his colleagues in OT and Speech were technically considered support services that were required by law to be available in the schools to help children reach their IEP goals, but he also felt very strongly about the professional duty he had to his young patients and he was not comfortable quite yet that he was meeting what he expected of himself as a licensed PT. The OT and Speech therapists were quite collegial but not much help, they seemed to passively accept what was in the IEP indicating to him that while they made recommendations often the final IEP was negotiated with the child's guardian with little input from the ancillary services. His predecessor in the position recently retired after many years in the district and while she left him a nice welcoming note, she did not provide any contact information. Scott's discomfort rose to a new level when he began to grapple with another issue, the four students who were not "coming to school in person." The district had given all of the parents the option to continue remote learning with the beginning of the fall semester if they were not comfortable sending their children back to school. Scott had four children whose IEP called for individual PT sessions twice a week, but they were not in school. Scott, thought treating children via telehealth was going to be a challenge but he felt comfortable with telehealth as a way to deliver care, having been immersed in it during the past year. What he wasn't prepared for was the realization that three of the four children were actually staying with family in other states, none of which Scott was licensed in and a quick check of the PT compact website, *PTcompact. org* revealed the states, were not yet part of the compact. Scott would not be able to use a Compact privilege to treat the children assigned to him and it could take months to secure the licenses he needed to treat these children. Scott contacted the Director of the Child Study Team to deliver the news and see what alternative plan could be made for the children. The Director calmly told Scott, he had nothing to worry about, the attorney for the district told him last year that it wasn't an issue because the children were registered in the school, and these were extraordinary times. Scott responded that he was aware that there were emergency orders in place during the pandemic that allowed for temporary licensure in other states but to his knowledge most of these had expired. The Director, glancing at his watch, and obviously in a hurry, reminded Scott that the attorney said it was fine, and the Director was also OK with Scott treating these children, after all Scott needed to realize that his role in a school setting was different than where he had been before. Scott took the cue, leaving the office, but not at all satisfied with the answer. He was quite cognizant of the fact that this was a new environment for him … but this setting, or for that matter any setting, did not absolve him of his personal professional responsibility or legal obligations … did it? Scott considered whether he should be comfortable accepting the advice of the attorney for the district, after all the attorney knows the law, and his colleagues seem ok with it, but on the other hand, it is Scott's license and his alone.

CONSIDER AND REFLECT

Scott is in a new setting. He understands there are some things he needs to learn but he also realizes that his understanding of his professional obligations and responsibilities are in conflict with others in his new work setting. He is being asked to undertake his job responsibilities in a way that did not make him feel comfortable both ethically or legally.

After working through the ethical decision-making process, what course of action would you suggest?

Ethical Decision-Making Worksheet

Case: _____

The Realm   Jack Glaser (1994)

Individual	Organizational/ Institutional	Societal
The good of the patient/ client and focuses on rights, duties, relationships and behaviors between individuals	Good of the organization, focuses on structures and systems, which facilitate organizational or institutional goals	Concerned with the common good

The Realm _____

Rationale:

The Individual Process: James Rest (1994, 1999)

Moral Sensitivity	Moral Judgment	Moral Motivation	Moral Courage	Moral Potency (Hannah and Avolio, 2010)
Recognizing, interpreting, and framing an ethical situation	Right versus wrong actions. Generating options, selecting and applying ethical principles	Priority on ethical values over other values. Professionalism is a primary motivator for ethical behavior	Implementing the chosen ethical action, development of a plan	Includes decision making that includes moral ownership, courage, and self-efficacy

The Individual Process: _____

Rationale:

The Situation   Swisher et al. (2005) adapted from Kidder

(continued on following page)

Issue/ Problem	Dilemma	Distress	Temptation	Silence
Important values present	Two alternative courses of action: Right vs. Right decision	The right course of action is known but the clinician cannot perform it	Choice between right and wrong	Values are challenged but no one is speaking about this challenge to values

The Situation: _____

Rationale:

_____

_____

_____

Ethical Principles and/or Standards of Ethical Conduct of the PTA (see Appendixes A and B)

Code of Ethics (Principles) for PTs	Rationale	Standards of Ethical Conduct (Standards) for PTAs	Rationale

Suggested Action:

CHAPTER 17

Supervision

Physical therapists (PTs) and physical therapist assistants (PTAs) are engaged in a variety of supervisory situations. The most important common factor that all types of supervision involve is the understanding that *delegation* does not in any way mean *abdication*. Licensed professionals are granted rights and expected to meet the obligations associated with their professional responsibility. PTs may be supervised by another individual, yet they must maintain professional independence in decision-making that benefits the patients they serve. All PTs have supervisory responsibilities when practicing in a setting that employs office help and aides as well as other PTs and PTAs. In addition, if a physical therapist has the opportunity to supervise students, another layer of supervision is encountered. Supervision can become very complex, with individuals having to answer to several supervisors simultaneously, for example, a supervisor for administrative duties and another for clinical practice. Communication is the key to good supervisor/supervisee relationships. An effective supervisor makes performance expectations clear and applies rules fairly and consistently. It is the responsibility of the supervisor to develop and maintain a supportive environment that all employees regardless of position are valued and treated with respect for their contributions to the organization.

Cases in this section:

Long-Distance Supervision	**Inappropriate supervision**
Supervision Revision	**Supervision conflict**
PRN PT or PTA	**Resisting supervision**
Supervisory Inaction	**Abuse of supervisory power**

Case Example 25

LONG-DISTANCE SUPERVISION
Inappropriate supervision

When we receive our license to practice, we are granted certain rights under the law, but we also have taken on certain responsibilities. It is imperative that we be familiar with and adhere to all dictates of the practice acts of states within which we work. To do otherwise is both illegal and unethical.

Sandra has been a physical therapist assistant (PTA) for 2 years. Her first job was at an outpatient clinic where a friend of hers was also employed, but she'd always wanted to work at a skilled nursing facility (SNF). When the opportunity arises to join a large company that owns SNFs in several states, she seeks out and secures a position. It strikes her as a perfect fit, in that she wants to serve older adults, the salary and benefits are better than they were in her old job, and she knows that she could at some point relocate within the same company if she so chooses.

In fact, one of the conditions of employment is that Sandra get licensed and be willing to substitute as needed at an SNF across the river, in a neighboring state from the facility at which she regularly works. She has no hesitation agreeing to this stipulation, as the other facility is only a 15-minute drive from her home.

Sandra is assigned to a small subacute facility in her home state for orientation and her first few months of employment. She quickly establishes a strong working relationship with Lori, her supervising physical therapist (PT). Lori is a wonderful and supportive teacher, and Sara thrives under her tutelage. About 4 months into their time together, Lori tells Sandra she'll be needed the following week at the SNF in the neighboring state, as someone there is going on vacation for a week. The news makes Sandra a little nervous, but Lori reminds her that she's been carrying her own caseload with supervision for months now and has done a good job. "You'll be fine!" Lori says, adding, "And you already know Tina."

Sandra doesn't really "know" Tina, the PT who'll be supervising her at the other facility, but she has met her a couple of times at meetings for area staff and has found her to be friendly and highly knowledgeable. So, the following Monday Sandra crosses over the bridge and confidently meets up with her new—if temporary—colleagues. Tina is very welcoming, as are Mike and Mabel, the aides to whom Sandra is introduced. Her first day goes smoothly, but Sandra is stunned when, in late afternoon, Tina says, "See, you fit right in here! I know I won't have to worry about you while I'm gone."

"Gone?" Sandra asks, suddenly worried and confused.

"My husband and I are off to Paris in the morning!" Tina says excitedly.

"But, who will be supervising me in your absence?" Sandra nervously asks.

"Direct supervision isn't required in this state," Tina says. "You'll be fine. And it's just for a few days."

Sandra realizes with a sinking feeling that she is subbing for a vacationing PT—not a vacationing PTA, as she had assumed. Sandra gets a chance before leaving that day to place a quick call to George, the company's regional administrator. He is not a PT, but he encourages staff to come to him with questions about company policies. George, who is based in Sandra's home state, confirms that supervision requirements are different "across the river." All Sandra needs to do, he says, is be able to communicate with a PT when and if it proves necessary.

"But my supervising PT is going to be in France!" Sandra blurts out. George tells her not to worry about it—just to take care of patients and leave the administrative details to others. Sandra is hardly reassured by George's words, as there won't be any other PT on staff at the facility while Tina is gone. Still, she figures she can ask Lori to countersign her patient notes and drive over to evaluate any new patients, since the distance is not prohibitive.

The next two days go well. There are no new patients, and Sandra enjoys working with the older adults she sees. Mike and Mable are able, helpful, and friendly. Sandra is a bit concerned that Lori hasn't yet come to countersign her patient notes, but she knows that Lori is busier than usual without Sandra there to assist her.

The following morning, however, Sandra learns that a new patient has arrived at the SNF overnight and needs to be evaluated. Mabel looks confused when Sandra says, "We can't do anything until I can get Lori over here for the evaluation."

"You mean you can't just do it yourself?" Mabel asks.

"I'm not totally familiar with this state's practice act, but no, I don't think so," Sandra responds.

She's finally able to reach Lori on the phone. Lori is surprised by and sympathetic to Sandra's dilemma—"I was under the impression you'd be subbing for a PTA," she says—but she adds that she's in no position either to countersign Sandra's notes or to conduct a patient evaluation at the neighboring facility.

"I'm not licensed to practice in that state," Lori says. "In fact, that's purposeful on my part. I don't need the headaches of the back-and-forth travel."

"What should I do?" Sandra asks.

"You need to get back in touch with George before you do anything else," Lori says. "Good luck. Let me know what happens."

They hang up, and Sandra begins to dial George's number. She is trying not to panic, but she finds it difficult to be calm as she reviews the facts. Lori can't help her. Tina is in Europe. Sandra can't find Tina's cell number on the company website, but will that phone even work overseas? And why had Mabel thought Sandra could perform the patient evaluation herself? Could that possibly be the case? Should she consult the state practice act before she even calls George? And why had George seemed so cavalier about the situation in their previous conversation?

CONSIDER AND REFLECT

Is there anyone not at fault in this scenario? What is the impact on patients who are being denied the full benefits of appropriate PT/PTA direction, supervision, and teamwork? Sandra is insufficiently familiar with the practice act of the state in which she is working. She knows what her home state's practice act requires of her, but she needs to be equally familiar with the practice act of the state in which she's currently working. Tina and Lori are guilty of ethical lapses and, surely, of practice act violations as well. George, while not himself a licensee, has a responsibility to see that practice act dictates are followed, and the letter of the law is followed. But the licensees—Sandra, Tina, and Lori—bear the ultimate responsibility.

After working through the ethical decision-making process, what course of action would you suggest?

Ethical Decision-Making Worksheet

Case: _____

The Realm   Jack Glaser (1994)

Individual	Organizational/ Institutional	Societal
The good of the patient/ client and focuses on rights, duties, relationships, and behaviors between individuals	Good of the organization, focuses on structures and systems, which facilitate organizational or institutional goals	Concerned with the common good

The Realm: _____

Rationale:

The Individual Process   James Rest (1994, 1999)

Moral Sensitivity	Moral Judgment	Moral Motivation	Moral Courage	Moral Potency (Hannah and Avolio, 2010)
Recognizing, interpreting, and framing an ethical situation	Right vs. wrong actions. Generating options, selecting and applying ethical principles	Priority on ethical values over other values. Professionalism is a primary motivator for ethical behavior	Implementing the chosen ethical action, development of a plan	Includes decision making that includes moral ownership, courage, and self-efficacy

The Individual Process: _____

Rationale:

The Situation   Swisher et al. (2005) adapted from Kidder

(continued on following page)

Issue/ Problem	Dilemma	Distress	Temptation	Silence
Important values present	Two alternative courses of action: Right vs. Right decision	The right course of action is known but the clinician cannot perform it	Choice between right and wrong	Values are challenged but no one is speaking about this challenge to values

The Situation: _____

Rationale:

Ethical Principles and/or Standards of Ethical Conduct of the PTA (see Appendixes A and B)

Code of Ethics (Principles) for PTs	Rationale	Standards of Ethical Conduct (Standards) for PTAs	Rationale

Suggested Action:

Case Example 26

SUPERVISION REVISION
Supervision conflict

The supervisory relationship between physical therapists (PTs) and physical therapist assistants (PTAs) is clearly defined in the Code of Ethics for the Physical Therapist and the Standards of Ethical Conduct for the

Physical Therapists Assistant, as well as by state law in most cases. But what can happen when one party crosses those lines and the other feels constrained by a power differential from restoring and reinforcing the proper boundaries?

Meryl and John have gotten to know each other through committee work for their state chapter of the APTA. Meryl is a PTA with eight years' clinical experience who has owned a small private outpatient clinic for the past five years. John is a PT with two years' experience who has been working in a hospital. John's first love is outpatient physical therapy, so, when Meryl—with whom he's developed a good rapport—offers him a job at a competitive salary with attractive benefits, he seizes the opportunity.

John has worked with PTAs but never before has had direct supervisory responsibility. Another twist to his new job is the fact that the practice owner—his boss—is a PTA. When he interviews, John asks Meryl the obvious questions about his role and her own. She assures him that while she has full administrative responsibility as practice owner, clinically she is a PTA—subject to all laws and ethical dictates governing PTA supervision.

The first two months on the job are all that John could've wished for. He finds his patient and client mix interesting, and he feels very comfortable working with Meryl in their respective clinical roles. After a while, however, John becomes aware that Meryl considers some longtime clients who stop in for physical therapy to be "established patients" who, in Meryl's view, needn't be evaluated by John. Her reasoning is that they initially were evaluated by John's predecessor. The problem with that, in John's view, is that some of those evaluations by a PT occurred a year or more ago.

When Meryl takes a day off to attend a ceremony at her son's college, John takes on two of these "established" patients. Reviewing their charts, he's surprised to discover that, in both cases, an initial evaluation recently was billed to insurance. John did not evaluate either patient. Looking further into the paperwork, he reads the evaluations. Both were signed by Meryl but lack his co-signature. John wonders if he's missing something. He's no expert on the law, he concedes. Surely Meryl wouldn't do anything illegal. Would she?

John starts reexamining in his mind some things to which he'd initially paid little heed, when he was busy adjusting to the new practices and procedures of the outpatient environment. While John has conducted the initial evaluation of every new patient, Meryl sometimes has tweaked plans of care without any discussion with him. She also has discharged patients without consulting him. On the other hand, however, John has found Meryl to be an excellent PTA—one whose considerable experience in the clinic is reflected in her knowledge, skills, and judgment. Has he been unduly influenced, John now asks himself, by his confidence in her and his belief that patients' needs are being met?

Meryl returns the next day, but there's a full patient load and John can't seem to find the right time to share his concerns. A week goes by. The workload eases slightly, but, still, John is hesitant to broach this touchy subject with the woman who signs his paychecks.

The following week, Meryl asks John to co-sign four sets of patient's notes. He's never met two of the individuals. It seems more than ever as if he and Meryl should have a frank discussion about supervision.

John stares down at the patient notes Meryl has left on his desk. To sign or not to sign? Perhaps, he thinks as he ponders the potential consequences of airing his concerns, the time for action isn't now, but rather at such time as Meryl's actions truly compromise patient care—should that day come.

CONSIDER AND REFLECT

While most jurisdictions permit PTA ownership of physical therapy practices and PTAs serving as administrative directors of clinics, all parties involved must make a concerted effort to recognize the uniqueness of the situation, ensure effective communication between ownership and PTs, and safeguard optimal (and legal) patient care. Scope of practice for PTs and scope of work for PTAs are governed by the same three-part criteria—skill set at entry level, regulatory parameters, and what the individual adds to his or her baseline skills over time. All three must be taken into account and considered in concert. In this scenario, Meryl's experience has deepened her competence, but that doesn't change her scope of practice or the regulatory requirements of her status as a PTA.

After working through the ethical decision-making process, what course of action would you suggest?

Ethical Decision-Making Worksheet

Case: _____

The Realm: Jack Glaser (1994)

Individual	Organizational/ Institutional	Societal
The good of the patient/ client and focuses on rights, duties, relationships, and behaviors between individuals	Good of the organization, focuses on structures and systems, which facilitate organizational or institutional goals	Concerned with the common good

(continued on following page)

The Realm: _____

Rationale:

The Individual Process   James Rest (1994, 1999)

Moral Sensitivity	Moral Judgment	Moral Motivation	Moral Courage	Moral Potency (Hannah and Avolio, 2010)
Recognizing, interpreting, and framing an ethical situation	Right vs. wrong actions. Generating options, selecting and applying ethical principles	Priority on ethical values over other values. Professionalism is a primary motivator for ethical behavior	Implementing the chosen ethical action, development of a plan	Includes decision making that includes moral ownership, courage, and self-efficacy

The Individual Process: _____

Rationale:

The Situation: Swisher et al. (2005) adapted from Kidder

Issue/ Problem	Dilemma	Distress	Temptation	Silence
Important values present	Two alternative courses of action: Right vs. Right decision	The right course of action is known but the clinician cannot perform it	Choice between right and wrong	Values are challenged but no one is speaking about this challenge to values

The Situation: _____

Rationale:

Ethical Principles and/or Standards of Ethical Conduct of the PTA (see Appendixes A and B)

Code of Ethics (Principles) for PTs	Rationale	Standards of Ethical Conduct (Standards) for PTAs	Rationale

(continued on following page)

Code of Ethics (Principles) for PTs	Rationale	Standards of Ethical Conduct (Standards) for PTAs	Rationale

Suggested Action:

Case Example 27

PRN PT OR PTA
Resisting supervision

Physical therapists (PTs) and physical therapist assistants (PTAs) work together as a team. A good relationship is essential with mutual trust and respect the foundation of the association. Together the team can be very powerful but that requires recognizing their strengths and limitations.

Mike started at Mountain View Rehab Services in September in upstate New York. The hospital specializes in head injury treatment and other neurological problems. He was anxious to settle into his new position and excited to be working with colleagues who shared his passion for working in an interprofessional environment with the complex patient population found at Mountain View. Mike shadowed Lynn, the department director, the first day and he was sure that he made the right choice in going to Mountain View. He couldn't wait to get his own caseload. Over the next few days, Mike began to pick up his own patients and was spending less time with Lynn during treatment hours, but she was more than willing to review patients and help him negotiate their complex electronic documentation system. Two weeks after he began, Mike was carrying a full caseload and was performing like he had been there for years. Lynn announced with Mike fully on board it was time to reorganize the teams. Each of the PTs worked directly with a PTA partner, and between the PT and PTA partner they shared a full caseload over the seven-day work week. When the PT partner was off, another PT was designated as supervisor, but the PTA was invaluable in carrying out the continuity of care for the established patients on program. Cadence was assigned to Mike, and he was quite pleased to have her as his partner. He noticed her right away, when he first came to Mountain View, thinking that she appeared more self-assured than some of the other PTAs. Mike had not worked with PTAs clinically previously, but he very much respected the role of the PTA and was looking forward to the type of teamwork this partnership arrangement would afford patients.

Cadence and Mike sat down right after lunch to discuss the caseload and how they would divide up the patients. Mike had spoken to Lynn about how supervision of PTAs occurred in the facility since treatment took place in different venues—the gym, the patients' rooms, other treatment areas for multi-disciplinary sessions. He had no doubt that Cadence would be comfortable without his close supervision, but he wanted to strike the right balance that would ensure optimal patient care. As the weeks went by, the pair fell into a good routine, and Mike was comfortable with what Cadence was doing but he did feel that she didn't always communicate with him as quickly as he would have preferred when there was a change in the patient's condition. Cadence told Mike "You worry too much! Believe me, if there was something you need to know I will let you know, I am really way more capable than you give me credit for." Mike spoke with Lynn, and she reassured him that Cadence really would keep him informed, and he should be grateful that he had a "self-starter" like Cadence to partner with. Mike relaxed a bit, but he still had that concern that he had the ultimate responsibility for the care of the patients that Cadence was treating. He wondered did he really have "a handle" on how the patients were doing after he completed the evaluation and Cadence stepped in? Mike's concerns were heightened one Monday morning when he went to see his new patient, Scott Mitchell. Cadence had provided the weekend coverage, so she was off on Friday and Monday. When Mike went to see Scott, he found that he had a cane and was up and walking around his room. Mike went to the nurse's station to find out how that had occurred. Mountain View had a very strict protocol that required a falls risk assessment by the physical therapy department prior to authorizing the patient to ambulate with an assistive device. Mike checked the roster and saw the admission from Sunday afternoon but did not see any documentation from the supervising PT, who happened to be Lynn, that Scott Mitchell was seen by her. Mike continued with his evaluation of Scott, and in their discussion, Scott reported that a young woman brought him the cane after she did "some of the stuff that Mike was doing with him now." Following his assessment Mike was concerned that Scott's stability was not sufficient to be cleared to walk with the cane he had been given.

He explained to Scott that until he could manage a little better, to be safe, he would have to use a walker. Mike was concerned as reflecting over the past few months there were other times when there was a program change that may appear to be beyond what Cadence should be doing as a PTA, but Mike was not sure just where to draw the line. Supervision of support personnel was new to him. When Cadence returned on Tuesday Mike asked her to set aside some time in the morning to talk. Mike asked Cadence for an explanation, specifically about her interaction with Scott Mitchell as issuing a cane required an evaluation, to Mike's understanding not in the scope of work of a PTA. Cadence confided in Mike that she is actually a PT, she took the NPTE for PT the six times permitted and hit the lifetime limit but was unable to pass the exam and could not take it again. New York permits PTs to take the NPTE for PTAs, and she passed that on the third try and was hired at Mountain View as a PTA, but she admits quite readily, she "thinks like a PT." How could she let Mr. Mitchell be confined to a wheelchair all night when she had the skills to evaluate him and give him his freedom? Mike is quite taken aback, he reviews the reason why he thought the choice of a cane was not a good one and Cadence retorted, that "it is a matter of opinion." Cadence is a PTA, but by her own admission she will "when necessary" function as a PT when it is in the best interest of the patient. She doesn't put Mike at ease when she leaves him with this parting statement. "You may try to take the girl out of PT but you can't take the PT out of the girl." Mike is uncertain what to do but knows initially he must make it clear to Cadence that this is not her judgment call. He is not confident that this discussion will be the end of it and Cadence will not cross the line in the future. He knows he has further obligations, but he is not quite sure what they are.

CONSIDER AND REFLECT

Mike accepts his responsibility to his patients and includes the responsibility to appropriately supervise PT support staff including a PTA. Cadence appears to have some difficulty reconciling her educational preparation with her regulatory limitations. What are the ethical responsibilities they both have?

Cadence was determined to be competent and licensed as a PTA and therefore needs to practice within the professional and regulatory scope of work for a PTA. What is Mike's responsibility if she consistently practices beyond the limits of her license? Mike has an additional concern. He did not agree with the falls assessment outcome that Cadence reported and her choice of assistive equipment for Mr. Mitchell makes him much more wary of how much supervision he needs to provide for Cadence. What do both clinicians have to consider in terms of their ethical relationship with each other?

After working through the ethical decision-making process, what course of action would you suggest?

Ethical Decision-Making Worksheet

Case: _____

The Realm   Jack Glaser (1994)

Individual	Organizational/ Institutional	Societal
The good of the patient/ client and focuses on rights, duties, relationships, and behaviors between individuals	Good of the organization, focuses on structures and systems, which facilitate organizational or institutional goals	Concerned with the common good

The Realm: _____

Rationale:

The Individual Process   James Rest (1994, 1999)

Moral Sensitivity	Moral Judgment	Moral Motivation	Moral Courage	Moral Potency (Hannah and Avolio, 2010)
Recognizing, interpreting, and framing an ethical situation	Right vs. wrong actions. Generating options, selecting and applying ethical principles	Priority on ethical values over other values. Professionalism is a primary motivator for ethical behavior	Implementing the chosen ethical action, development of a plan	Includes decision making that includes moral ownership, courage, and self-efficacy

The Individual Process: _____

Rationale:

The Situation   Swisher et al. (2005) adapted from Kidder

Issue/ Problem	Dilemma	Distress	Temptation	Silence
Important values present	Two alternative courses of action: Right vs. Right decision	The right course of action is known but the clinician cannot perform it	Choice between right and wrong	Values are challenged but no one is speaking about this challenge to values

(continued on following page)

The Situation: _____

Rationale:

Ethical Principles and/or Standards of Ethical Conduct of the PTA (see Appendixes A and B)

Code of Ethics (Principles) for PTs	Rationale	Standards of Ethical Conduct (Standards) for PTAs	Rationale

Suggested Action:

Case Example 28

SUPERVISORY INACTION
Abuse of supervisory power

Supervisory inaction
There is always a delicate balance between work and the demands of personal life. While we all try to achieve a perfect work life balance, there are many factors that impact that ideal. Sometimes the stress of either work or home, or both results in ethical risk factors, situations that result in poor decisions that under other circumstances would not happen.

Abuse of supervisory power
Tom is a physical therapist assistant, (PTA) at Holly Hills, a large subacute facility with head trauma, memory care, and respirator

dependent units in addition to all of the standard services. PT, OT, and Speech work very closely together. The facility is currently expanding and as part of that expansion the Rehab common treatment area has been significantly decreased so most of the treatment is occurring on the floors with occasional treatment occurring in the commons as the rehab staff calls the joint treatment area. Tom and his colleagues miss the camaraderie that they enjoyed when they treated in the same space. It seems to Tom that there have been so many changes impacting patient care over the past two years, a pandemic, payment changes, productivity requirements and now this change in culture where most treatment is bedside. Tom and all of his colleagues seem to be constantly trying to adapt to new requirements, and to balance those demands with providing the excellent standard of care they are accustomed to providing. Now they realize how much they were missing not being able to collaborate with one another. At lunch Tom and his supervising PT Chrissy usually plan to eat together. She seems distracted and Tom is concerned that something may be bothering her, but he doesn't want to intrude. Chrissy seems to realize that Tom is quietly sitting at the table and focuses on him for a moment and then speaks, "Sorry Tom, I am lost in my own world today, I don't mean to be rude." Tom assures Chrissy that he totally understands, there is a lot going on lately, and asks is there anything I can do? Chrissy shares with Tom that she is worried, her wife's job has changed and now she has to leave by 6 which is great for the afternoon pickup but that leaves the morning chaos of getting the kids off to school to her. Tom doesn't have kids, but he can just imagine what mornings must be like. General supervision is permitted where they practice so Tom is completely comfortable telling Chrissy, not to worry about it, there is a simple solution. Normally they review the schedule in the morning and discuss any patients that they think they should confer about. They could take a look at the schedule the night before and discuss the patients on the morning schedule that way he can get started, and if he had any questions, she is just a phone call away. Chrissy seemed relieved but still seemed concerned. The new schedule started the following week and Tom and Chrissy easily adapted to their schedule and actually found it to be a very efficient plan as they reviewed the day and planned for the next day. Chrissy seemed much more relaxed, she was usually in by 8:30 at the latest and she managed to get her patients treated, the only difference Tom could see was that her schedule contained at least one co-treat per day, which was not something that Chrissy normally liked to do. Several weeks after they started this new schedule Tom was approached by Mandy the rehab director shortly after 8 asking if he knew where Chrissy was. Tom was pretty noncommittal, just saying, "I am not sure where she is right now." He did not mention it to Chrissy, though he did find it strange that Mandy was only concerned about where Chrissy was and no one else. Chrissy actually initiated the discussion a few days later when she came to Tom to tell him that Mandy called her in to her office to tell her that even though she is meeting her productivity numbers she is logging in 20–30 minutes late every day, and that has to change. Tom can see the panic in Chrissy's eyes. The co-workers wonder why it should make a difference if she is treating her patients and her outcomes are good and she is supervising Tom appropriately, why should it be a concern? Chrissy sighs and is resigned to try to come up with a solution that can get her to work on time. The next two days Chrissy makes it right on time without a minute to spare, her sister was able to help her out, but she is going to be on her own again. The next morning she is late and Tom sees her at lunch and she looks very stressed, she is almost in tears explaining to Tom, "I am a good PT, I am doing a good job with my patients, when I am here I am 150% on board, I just need a little flexibility," She hands Tom a piece of paper and says, "please hang on to this, it is my password, I know I should never share it but I am desperate, if it looks like I may be late, I am going to ask you to log me in, obviously I won't bill or document if I am not here but I don't have another choice." She doesn't give Tom a moment to respond, leaving the room to go treat her next patient. Tom is clearly uncomfortable, putting the paper in his pocket, hoping that this will be resolved another way. The next few days are fine, and Tom is hopeful that the issue is resolved but on Friday he gets a desperate text from Chrissy, "Hey Tom, sign me in please I will be there really soon." He sees Mandy at the computer terminal and pretty sure she is checking log in status he quickly grabs the paper and before he can reconsider, he logs Chrissy in. He walks away feeling very uncomfortable and wondering if anyone else is aware of what he has done, and now that he has done it once … will he be expected to do it again …. Will it become the expected practice?

CONSIDER AND REFLECT

Tom and Chrissy have a good professional relationship however because of personal pressures she has asked her colleague, over whom she has supervisory responsibility, to do something for her that compromises his ethical standards, yet, he feels little power to refuse her request. The ethical questions this situation raises are for both Tom and Chrissy. Chrissy's actions compromise her integrity and place her colleague in a similar position. Her actions may have been dictated by ethical risk factors. Tom's, the result of her actions, are complicated by the power gradient that exists between Chrissy and Tom.

After working through the ethical decision-making process, what course of action would you suggest?

Ethical Decision-Making Worksheet

Case: _____

The Realm   Jack Glaser (1994)

Individual	Organizational/Institutional	Societal
The good of the patient/client and focuses on rights, duties, relationships and behaviors between individuals	Good of the organization, focuses on structures and systems, which facilitate organizational or institutional goals	Concerned with the common good

The Realm _____

Rationale:

The Individual Process: James Rest (1994, 1999)

Moral Sensitivity	Moral Judgment	Moral Motivation	Moral Courage	Moral Potency (Hannah and Avolio, 2010)
Recognizing, interpreting, and framing an ethical situation	Right versus wrong actions. Generating options, selecting and applying ethical principles	Priority on ethical values over other values. Professionalism is a primary motivator for ethical behavior	Implementing the chosen ethical action, development of a plan	Includes decision making that includes moral ownership, courage, and self-efficacy

The Individual Process: _____

Rationale:

The Situation   Swisher et al. (2005) adapted from Kidder

Issue/Problem	Dilemma	Distress	Temptation	Silence
Important values present	Two alternative courses of action: Right vs. Right decision	The right course of action is known but the clinician cannot perform it	Choice between right and wrong	Values are challenged but no one is speaking about this challenge to values

(continued on following page)

The Situation: _____

Rationale:

_____

_____

_____

Ethical Principles and/or Standards of Ethical Conduct of the PTA (see Appendixes A and B)

Code of Ethics (Principles) for PTs	Rationale	Standards of Ethical Conduct (Standards) for PTAs	Rationale

Suggested Action:

CHAPTER 18

The Student Physical Therapist

There is both an art and a science to the delivery of healthcare. The safe and effective healthcare practitioner must become capable in both aspects of care. Throughout history, the education of each generation of healthcare providers is the responsibility of those already engaged in the practice of the profession. This results in certain unique challenges for both the provider and the novice learning to acquire the skills necessary to provide care. There is benefit obviously to the student in their clinical education, but there is also benefit to the facility and clinicians that provide the clinical education. The student in the clinical setting has unique ethical and legal ramifications. The student is not licensed, yet through their relationship with their clinical instructor they are responsible to adhere to all of the legal requirements of the jurisdiction in which they are practicing. They are also responsible to adhere to the Code of Ethics/ or Standards of Ethical Conduct of the American Physical Therapy Association. All of this occurs within the context of both the facility where they are placed and their academic institution. It is easy to understand how the student can find themselves at times conflicted regarding their responsibility. While they may understand and appreciate their role as they develop into an entry-level practitioner, they are responsible to fulfill that role under the supervision of their clinical instructor. The cases in this section highlight some of the different ways in which the relationship between the student and the clinical instructor (CI) may be challenged.

When physical therapists (PTs) and physical therapist assistants (PTAs) agree to work with a student, they take on a significant responsibility, but there are many positive benefits of the student–clinical instructor relationship, and competence is one of them. Helping a new clinician become competent is rewarding, and nobody can deny the professional growth that a clinical instructor experiences as a result of their mentorship role. The clinical instructor and the student both have the responsibility to maintain a positive learning environment while never losing sight of their shared responsibility to the patient.

Cases in this section:

Student or PT	Abdication of supervision
The Student Advocate	New professional responsibility
Project Professional Skills	Inappropriate professional behavior
See Some Evil?	Whose duty to report?

Case Example 29

STUDENT OR PT?
Abdication of supervision

Bob considers himself very fortunate; his first clinical placement following the conclusion of his first year in PT school has been an incredible
experience. His CI Stephanie, the practice manager, has been welcoming
and willing to share not just her PT knowledge but insights into the business of physical therapy. In addition to her position as practice manager,
Stephanie was one of the PTs for a dance troupe based in the city, but she
accompanied them for two weeks at a time twice a year when they went
on tour. Stephanie explained to Bob that she would be leaving on tour,
but fortunately it was during the final two weeks of his clinical placement.
Bob wasn't quite sure why that was fortunate, but he trusted that Stephanie
had the whole situation under control. He was determined to get as much
as he could out of the next few weeks before Stephanie left; he kidded her
that now that he knew she was leaving "he planned to drain her brain." The
Friday before she left she sat down with Bob to review his performance.
She was very complimentary of his performance at this point and told him
that she was confident that the next two weeks would be most beneficial
as he gained confidence in his skills. The PTA Gail could help him out if
he needed it; they would not be admitting any new patients, and Tim, the
agency float PT, would be in for two to three days per week depending on
the caseload at the other offices. Stephanie had demonstrated through all
of her interactions that she was a very knowledgeable practitioner, and Bob
was confident that what he would be doing must be OK. Even though he
was pretty sure he was supposed to be supervised, he was never completely
clear about what exactly supervision is meant to happen—after all since
week four, Stephanie was always available but not always right by his side.
Bob was actually quite excited that his CI was confident in his ability to
carry on in her absence, allowing him to rely on his skills, and he still had
staff to rely on. Gail had been a PTA for a long time and Tim the float PT
was used to fitting in to operations that were up and running. Stephanie
was careful to make sure that Bob knew all of the patients, and he was
clear on the plan of care. She left him Tim's phone number "just in case."
The first two days Bob was quite comfortable—he continued the plan of
care that he helped Stephanie create before she left, and he felt pretty confident. He accepted that his documentation would await the arrival of Tim
who would countersign his notes. He prepared the billing forms the way
Stephanie showed him, giving little thought to whose license number that
billing form was utilizing, or the fact that he was billing Medicare Part B,
something that he vaguely recollected was "not permitted." On the third

day, Bob had a wake-up call. A patient he had been treating arrived in considerable pain. Bob immediately went to Gail who suggested that he give Tim a call. Tim responded right away, but not knowing the patient he suggested that Bob tell the patient that he cannot treat him and he should call his doctor. The patient was visibly annoyed, stating he has had this type of a flare up before, and it always calmed down with some stretching and that machine that makes you skin tingly. Bob knew he could do what the patient was telling him "works," but he was not sure why there was pain and he recognized that "just because he could, didn't mean he should." Bob was conflicted; he wanted to do what was best for the patient, but he just wasn't sure what was the best thing to do.

The incident was a "wake-up call" for Bob. Confronted with a patient in pain, his first instinct was to provide the care that the patient requested; however, he recognized that his limited experience should make him apprehensive. He suddenly saw that perhaps his ego had gotten danger-ously in the way of his judgment.

CONSIDER AND REFLECT

If Stephanie hasn't quite "created a monster" in Bob, she's certainly encouraged him—through her supervisory, billing, and perhaps other practices—to be "flex-ible" with the rules of legal and ethical conduct. She's fed his ego and praised his "instincts"—but those instincts now are at odds. To treat Dan, or to step back? To trust Stephanie on billing matters, or ask Tim for feedback, after all? What's in the patient's best interest?

After working through the ethical decision-making process, what course of action would you suggest?

Ethical Decision-Making Worksheet

Case: _____

The Realm   Jack Glaser (1994)

Individual	Organizational/ Institutional	Societal
The good of the patient/client and focuses on rights, duties, relationships, and behaviors between individuals	Good of the organization, focuses on structures and systems, which facilitate organizational or institutional goals	Concerned with the common good

(continued on following page)

The Realm: _____

Rationale:

The Individual Process   James Rest (1994, 1999)

Moral Sensitivity	Moral Judgment	Moral Motivation	Moral Courage	Moral Potency (Hannah and Avolio, 2010)
Recognizing, interpreting, and framing an ethical situation	Right vs. wrong actions. Generating options, selecting and applying ethical principles	Priority on ethical values over other values. Professionalism is a primary motivator for ethical behavior	Implementing the chosen ethical action, development of a plan	Includes decision making that includes moral ownership, courage, and self-efficacy

The Individual Process: _____

Rationale:

The Situation   Swisher et al. (2005) adapted from Kidder

Issue/ Problem	Dilemma	Distress	Temptation	Silence
Important values present	Two alternative courses of action: Right vs. Right decision	The right course of action is known but the clinician cannot perform it	Choice between right and wrong	Values are challenged but no one is speaking about this challenge to values

The Situation: _____

Rationale:

Ethical Principles and/or Standards of Ethical Conduct of the PTA (see Appendixes A and B)

Code of Ethics (Principles) for PTs	Rationale	Standards of Ethical Conduct (Standards) for PTAs	Rationale

(continued on following page)

Code of Ethics (Principles) for PTs	Rationale	Standards of Ethical Conduct (Standards) for PTAs	Rationale

Suggested Action:

Case Example 30

THE STUDENT ADVOCATE
New professional responsibility

Patient and client advocacy isn't always easy, and sometimes it puts us at odds with others, but our professional ethics require it. Consider the following scenario involving a student and her clinical instructor (CI).

Meghan is in the final year of her Doctor of Physical Therapy (DPT) program and midway through her second full-tie clinical rotation. She enjoys the challenges of working in a busy outpatient clinic at a local hospital and feels fortunate to have an excellent CI. Ken is a dedicated PT who is only five years out of school himself and plans to seek specialty certification in cardiovascular and pulmonary physical therapy.

Today's first patient is Allison, a self-referral. The petite thirty-one-year-old reports neck pain and reduced range of motion in her neck and shoulders. Ken takes the lead because Allison's presentation is somewhat unusual in a patient so young. He instructs Meghan to take note of the types of questions he asks during his examination and how he employs his clinical reasoning skills during evaluation.

Something in Allison's paperwork suggests a traumatic precipitating incident. She seems very shy and is a poor presenter of her medical history. When Ken asks her if she has had neck pain in the past, for example, she doesn't answer immediately, then tentatively nods, "Yes." When Ken asks how long ago that was, she shrugs slightly and says, "Maybe last year. I'm not sure." Subsequent medical questions are met with similar vagueness. Allison volunteers that she had worked as a secretary until about six months ago but is not currently employed. She and her husband, Ralph, have no children, she says. She twice miscarried, she adds softly, looking down at the floor.

Ken examines her neck and shoulders and confirms the issues Allison has reported. She says she can't recall any particular incident that might have caused the pain and tightness. "Nothing?" Ken asks. Allison again shrugs slightly. But then she says, "I feel a little stressed sometimes when Ralph gets home from work, and something went wrong at the plant that day. He's a good man, but he drinks when he's upset and he can have a pretty bad temper." Unnerved by that statement, Meghan shoots Ken a look. But he is gazing dispassionately down at his notes.

Looking back up at Allison, Ken says, "Let's see if some of this pain is related to your posture. Oh, and by the way, do you see a dentist regularly? Sometimes people have what's called 'referred pain' from gum infections or other dental issues." He continues the examination, still seeking a definitive diagnosis. When he asks Allison to stand so he can check her posture, Ken and Meghan notice at the same moment an area of discoloration on her right shoulder. Seeing where their eyes are turned, Allison says sheepishly, "I dropped a jar in the kitchen and Ralph yanked me away so I wouldn't step on the shards. He's a lot bigger than I am and sometimes he doesn't know his own strength."

That account makes Meghan even more uneasy about what she feels may be the real source of Allison's pain. She is certain that this time Ken will follow up. She waits for him to ask additional questions to prompt Allison to elaborate, and to signal that this is a safe environment in which she can speak openly. To Meghan's surprise, however, Ken completes his evaluation without saying a word about the dropped-jar story. He instructs Allison in a basic home-exercise program, then directs her to the front desk to make an appointment for later that week.

It's a very busy day in the clinic, and for several hours Meghan can't find an appropriate time to voice her concerns to Ken. Nor is she entirely certain she should, as she doesn't want to be seen as challenging his judgment. At the end of the work day, however, Ken gives her a slight opening when he remarks, "Crazy day, huh?"

"Crazy," Meghan agrees. "It was a little weird. Like, you know, I was thinking about what our first patient, Allison said about her husband. Do you think there's any chance her pain could be caused by spousal abuse?"

Ken laughs slightly, "What, because old Ralph has a temper sometimes? I appreciate the fact that you're concerned, but a lot of husbands fit that description. Besides, if he's such a bad guy, why didn't he pick her up and set her down on that broken glass instead of pulling her away from it?"

Meghan can't believe what she's hearing! Ken always has struck her as being caring and compassionate, but he clearly isn't even slightly skeptical of the dropped-jar story. She's trying to decide what to say next when he notes the surprise on her face and cajoles her, "C'mon. I think we need a little more to go on than that, okay?"

Meghan nods, realizing that the discussion is over as far as Ken's concerned. But she can't get Allison out of her head. The next morning, she calls her director of clinical education (DCE), seeking his counsel. She recounts the entire story and says, "I feel that we should be advocating for this patient, but I'm not sure what to do. I know from our legal issues class that under state law we're supposed to report suspected abuse of children and senior citizens. But what about suspected abuse of people at in-between ages?"

Her DCE confirms that state law doesn't directly address reporting suspected abuse of non-senior adults, but he adds, "Your instinct to help is appropriate. How about this: I'll email you a list of websites tonight to share with this patient—an abuse hotline and some social services resources she can contact if she wants to. Give it to her the next time she comes into the clinic. Just say, 'In case you need this,' or something like that. You don't have to make a big deal. But it will not only give her information she might need, but will convey to her that somebody is listening, if she needs that message. And that's important."

Meghan feels better about the situation by the day of Allison's second appointment. She has in the pocket of her lab coat a printout of the information her DCE had emailed her and is prepared to hand it to Allison before she leaves. But Allison never arrives. "Seems that we've got a no-show," Ken says, simply. Recalling that Allison had been a self-referral, Meghan now wonders if the first visit had been a cry for help. Perhaps she decided to give up after Ken dismissed her provocative statements.

Meghan feels she must make another attempt to share with Ken her concerns. She shows him the printout and asks if perhaps one of them should reach out to Allison over the phone. Ken sighs and responds, "You know my feelings about this. But if you want to make that call, be my guest." He hands Meghan Allison's chart, on which her phone number is written.

Although she's a bit concerned that this disagreement might adversely affect her relationship with Ken, Meghan looks him in the eye and says, "I think I will call her, then. Thanks." Ken simply nods. As she leaves the room, she feels good about her decision. She's eager to share with Allison the information she's gathered, and she hopes to convince her to return to physical therapy.

CONSIDER AND REFLECT

As a student, Meghan's instinct is to defer to her CI's experience and expertise. She yields instead to the higher calling of patient advocacy, while recognizing the importance of consultation and transparency in the process. Providing resources to patients or clients who we believe are seeking our help is part of our role as patient and client advocates and our responsibility as ethical practitioners. Following up with patients or clients with whom we've established a professional relationship is important for continuity of care, as well. Students are encouraged and expected to check in with their school when situations arise that give them discomfort and raise questions.

After working through the ethical decision-making process, what course of action would you suggest?

Ethical Decision-Making Worksheet

Case: _____

The Realm: Jack Glaser (1994)

Individual	Organizational/ Institutional	Societal
The good of the patient/ client and focuses on rights, duties, relationships, and behaviors between individuals	Good of the organization, focuses on structures and systems, which facilitate organizational or institutional goals	Concerned with the common good

The Realm: _____

Rationale:

The Individual Process   James Rest (1994, 1999)

Moral Sensitivity	Moral Judgment	Moral Motivation	Moral Courage	Moral Potency (Hannah and Avolio, 2010)
Recognizing, interpreting, and framing an ethical situation	Right vs. wrong actions. Generating options, selecting and applying ethical principles	Priority on ethical values over other values. Professionalism is a primary motivator for ethical behavior	Implementing the chosen ethical action, development of a plan	Includes decision making that includes moral ownership, courage, and self-efficacy

(continued on following page)

The Individual Process: _____

Rationale:

The Situation: Swisher et al. (2005) adapted from Kidder

Issue/ Problem	Dilemma	Distress	Temptation	Silence
Important values present	Two alternative courses of action: Right vs. Right decision	The right course of action is known but the clinician cannot perform it	Choice between right and wrong	Values are challenged but no one is speaking about this challenge to values

The Situation: _____

Rationale:

Ethical Principles and/or Standards of Ethical Conduct of the PTA
(see Appendixes A and B)

Code of Ethics (Principles) for PTs	Rationale	Standards of Ethical Conduct (Standards) for PTAs	Rationale

Suggested Action:

Case Example 31

PROJECT PROFESSIONAL SKILLS
Inappropriate professional behavior

Students look forward to their clinical rotations as an opportunity to develop and refine their clinical skills. They don't necessarily consider that their professional skills are also part of the developmental process and equally important in the safe and effective care of a patient.

Margie is an experienced clinical instructor, having had many students from a variety of universities. She loves watching them develop their clinical skills and confidence and enjoys their enthusiasm and passion. Kelsey, her newest student, is a third-year student in her last clinical rotation. This is her first acute care affiliation and although she was assigned to the placement she wanted, she is pretty sure that acute care is not for her and has made Margie aware of that. Kelsey made it clear that she is focused twelve weeks ahead when she will be done and off across the country to what she hopes will be her ideal job in an outpatient setting. The first two days Kelsey was on time, but by the middle of the week she started getting to the hospital on time but once she parked and got to PT she was late. Margie was concerned, but Kelsey came in ready to hit the ground running and appeared to have a reasonable excuse each time for her tardiness. Kelsey was a quick learner; it was apparent that she was a strong student and while she did not appear to be particularly engaged in the acute care setting, she was not intimidated, and she was providing an acceptable level of care. What was of concern to Margie was while the care was acceptable, it was not at the level she thought it could be. Kelsey appeared to just provide the minimum; what was more of concern was that Kelsey exhibited some behaviors and biases that she saw no problem with and almost seemed cavalier in her attitude toward some of the patients. Over the first few weeks Margie ignored some of the side comments about patients' weight and gender and religious preferences. She was giving Kelsey the benefit of the doubt and allowing her a little leeway as she became acclimated. Finally, one Thursday afternoon Margie felt she had been pushed to her limit. Kelsey had been coming in late every day and when approached about it indicated that "she was always ready to treat, isn't that what really matters?" Kelsey met Margie at the nurses' station that morning and loudly stated that she was unable to see Mr. Myers because "he was out of it for a change, and quite honestly he doesn't benefit from PT, it is a waste of her time." Margie was shocked, but with her usual calm demeanor she decided to try to get a better understanding of Kelsey's reasoning. Kelsey was quite willing to share, clearly stating that Mr. Myers, like so many of the other patients on this general medical floor, didn't really "need" PT.

He was just too sick and too old to really benefit, and by treating him will take away much needed services from other patients like the athletes on the orthopedic floor who really benefit from PT. Margie began to piece together a disturbing trend. Kelsey often cancelled the patients on the General Medical floor for a variety of reasons and spent the time on the orthopedic floor. She also cut sessions short claiming the patient was too tired or was confused. Twice she told Margie Mrs. Rivera was not available and made an offhand comment about "illegals" getting all the medical care they needed while "hard-working Americans were denied treatment." Margie had ignored the comments thinking it was a rather lame attempt at humor, hadn't Kelsey read Mrs. Rivera's chart? She was a retired principal from the local middle school. Margie thought about it overnight, and the next morning before they started seeing patients, she pulled Kelsey aside and told her she was concerned about her attitude toward some of the patients and felt it was detrimental to her relationship with her patients and it appeared to be affecting her plan of care. Kelsey seemed surprised and a little defensive, explaining to Margie that she thought she had a responsibility to determine who needed care and who did not based on her evaluation. Margie did not deny that it was a professional responsibility to determine the plan of care, but it wasn't just the clinical findings that had to be considered. Kelsey responded that she knew that she wanted to provide PT only for people who really needed it, and should be entitled to receive it, the exact reason she was planning to relocate and work in an outpatient setting upon graduation!

Margie could not deny that clinically Kelsey's skills were at entry level, but her professional behaviors were alarming—she was disrespectful and had biases that while she attempted to cover them up with well-crafted excuses were of great concern. Her ongoing discussions with Kelsey did little to change her behavior over the course of the affiliation, and Margie was not sure if she should report her concerns to the school, beyond that which is captured by the Clinical Performance Instrument (CPI). The responsibility to graduate a competent, safe, and effective practitioner lies ultimately with the school, but the academic institution must rely on the clinical sites to report situations to them that impact the student's ability to achieve entry-level competence.

CONSIDER AND REFLECT

Margie is concerned that her future colleague Kelsey has the clinical ability to be a therapist, but her professional behaviors, certainly more difficult to measure, are of great concern and do have a significant impact on practice. Kelsey treated patients differently, and was based on her comments there appeared to be evidence of bias.

Margie knew it would be extremely difficult to effectively describe the very troubling behaviors she observed other than the tardiness. Kelsey's lack of cultural sensitivity, her discriminatory tendencies all clearly affect her clinical decision making and her professional judgment.

After working through the ethical decision-making process, what course of action would you suggest?

Ethical Decision-Making Worksheet

Case: _____

The Realm   Jack Glaser (1994)

Individual	Organizational/ Institutional	Societal
The good of the patient/ client and focuses on rights, duties, relationships, and behaviors between individuals	Good of the organization, focuses on structures and systems, which facilitate organizational or institutional goals	Concerned with the common good

The Realm: _____

Rationale:

The Individual Process   James Rest (1994, 1999)

Moral Sensitivity	Moral Judgment	Moral Motivation	Moral Courage	Moral Potency (Hannah and Avolio, 2010)
Recognizing, interpreting, and framing an ethical situation	Right vs. wrong actions. Generating options, selecting and applying ethical principles	Priority on ethical values over other values. Professionalism is a primary motivator for ethical behavior	Implementing the chosen ethical action, development of a plan	Includes decision making that includes moral ownership, courage, and self-efficacy

(continued on following page)

The Individual Process: _____

Rationale:

The Situation   Swisher et al. (2005) adapted from Kidder

Issue/ Problem	Dilemma	Distress	Temptation	Silence
Important values present	Two alternative courses of action: Right vs. Right decision	The right course of action is known but the clinician cannot perform it	Choice between right and wrong	Values are challenged but no one is speaking about this challenge to values

The Situation: _____

Rationale:

Ethical Principles and/or Standards of Ethical Conduct of the PTA
(see Appendixes A and B)

Code of Ethics (Principles) for PTs	Rationale	Standards of Ethical Conduct (Standards) for PTAs	Rationale

Suggested Action:

Case Example 32

SEE SOME EVIL?
Whose duty to report?

Gary was excited to begin his last full time clinical rotation in a large out patient facility. Though he enjoyed all his placements so far this is the one he really had the highest expectations for. He has been hearing about Apex PT through social media and even advertised on the radio. He knew it to be by reputation fast paced and state of the art, both which appealed to him in every way. While very popular with the young sports crowd the practice treated adults of all ages and he looked forward to seeing how they managed the various patient populations in the same physical environment. His CI Holly had been at Apex for four years but had experience before that in several other out patient environments, he could tell immediately he was going to learn a lot with her guidance. The first two days Gary basically tagged after Holly … you might say at a rather high paced run. She explained that it took organization and planning to be successful at Apex but he would catch on quickly. She had two evaluation slots per day that were thirty-minute individual time periods and in her other treatment hours she had five patients scheduled. She was supported by four assigned aides. She expected by the end of the rotation he would be able to manage the evaluations on her case load and at least four patients an hour of course supported by the aides and one group session. Quick and efficient thinking and problem solving was the hallmark of effective care at Apex. It did not take long for Gary to acclimate to the pace and the well-trained aides certainly helped him to move his patients along, but Gary had a nagging thought that perhaps the care was not as effective as it could be. Patients seemed to be on schedule longer than he had seen at other places both as a student and as an aide. He also, in all of his years of being an aide never had been given the amount of responsibility these aides were. He agreed they were well-trained, but he wondered not if they were practicing beyond their scope, he knew, they didn't have a scope, what he wondered was why they could practice so differently at Apex than any place else he had been. Gary rose to the challenge and shortly after midterm he assumed a full entry level therapist caseload and was managing the supervision and documentation challenges that came with practice. Concurrent with his final placement he was completing his business practice elective and he asked Holly if she could spare a little time to review the billing process with him, the one piece that still stymied him. Holly was happy to set up some time with the billing group so he could see what happened after he submitted the paperwork that generated the final bill. He was not quite sure exactly how his documentation in the electronic medical record generated the final bill but he was looking forward to connecting all of the dots. The appointment with the biller was early in the morning before his first patient arrived. When he met up with Holly he admitted to her that he was probably more confused about the whole billing thing than he was before he met with the biller. Holly welcomed him to the club and said that is why it is all about "codes" it is a mystery to us all, but the bills get generated, processed and the patients seem ok with it all …. So he should just be glad all he has to do is make it clear enough in the paper to answer the questions and be happy he doesn't have to do the billing. Gary considered his CI's advice but something was just making him feel a bit uncomfortable. He recalled in his Administration and Management class learning that billing was his responsibility, it was a part of his practice, he recalled having it pointed out in the law that he had the responsibility to manage all aspects of the patients care, and his responsibility included accurate documentation and billing of the services provided and he remembered also that Principle 7E required him to be aware of charges and ensure "that documentation and coding for physical therapy services accurately reflect the nature and extent of services provided." Gary reflected on the two bills he saw. One for a patient with private insurance billed for sixty minutes of skilled PT services. Gary saw the patient for ten minutes of that sixty minutes billed. Aides under his direction managed the care for the rest of the time. The other patient had Medicare and was billed for sixty minutes also, but Gary was well aware that he with the aides saw that patient in a group. Gary was acutely aware he was a student, weeks away from graduation, was this the time to question what he was seeing, his CI is a great PT surely there is an explanation for what he is seeing that explains what appear to be some billing inconsistencies. Gary learned that we have a duty to report … but surely everyone around him is aware and can explain these billing irregularities … for now it is probably best to adopt that old "go along to get along" adage.

CONSIDER AND REFLECT

Students often find themselves in a difficult position. They may observe behaviors or actions that they are aware are inappropriate yet it is difficult to take action. For anyone it would require moral courage for a student who feels very vulnerable it would require moral potency to take action. Students need to be empowered just like clinicians to take ownership of their actions. Students who do take action report issues of concern to their Director of Clinical Education. Safeguards are in place so that a student who has the moral courage to report is not adversely impacted. The responsibility of what to do with the information has now been shifted to the licensed physical therapist the DCE. The DCE must take action (even inaction is an action) and knows the action may have an impact on the University, future students and of course the profession. In these difficult situations, rationalization may be the easier course to take until we remind ourselves that "there is never a right way to do the wrong thing." (adapted from Mark Twain).

After working through the ethical decision-making process, what course of action would you suggest?

Ethical Decision-Making Worksheet

Case: _____

The Realm   Jack Glaser (1994)

Individual	Organizational/ Institutional	Societal
The good of the patient/ client and focuses on rights, duties, relationships and behaviors between individuals	Good of the organization, focuses on structures and systems, which facilitate organizational or institutional goals	Concerned with the common good

The Realm _____

Rationale:

The Individual Process: James Rest (1994, 1999)

Moral Sensitivity	Moral Judgment	Moral Motivation	Moral Courage	Moral Potency (Hannah and Avolio, 2010)
Recognizing, interpreting, and framing an ethical situation	Right versus wrong actions. Generating options, selecting and applying ethical principles	Priority on ethical values over other values. Professionalism is a primary motivator for ethical behavior	Implementing the chosen ethical action, development of a plan	Includes decision making that includes moral ownership, courage, and self-efficacy

(continued on following page)

The Individual Process: _____

Rationale:

The Situation   Swisher et al. (2005) adapted from Kidder

Issue/ Problem	Dilemma	Distress	Temptation	Silence
Important values present	Two alternative courses of action: Right vs. Right decision	The right course of action is known but the clinician cannot perform it	Choice between right and wrong	Values are challenged but no one is speaking about this challenge to values

The Situation: _____

Rationale: _____
_____
_____

Ethical Principles and/or Standards of Ethical Conduct of the PTA (see Appendixes A and B)

Code of Ethics (Principles) for PTs	Rationale	Standards of Ethical Conduct (Standards) for PTAs	Rationale

Suggested Action:

Code of Ethics for the Physical Therapist

HOD S06-20-28-25 [Amended HOD S06-19-47-67; HOD S06-09-07-12; HOD S06-00-12-23; HOD 06-91-05-05; HOD 06-87-11-17; HOD 06-81-06-18; HOD 06-78-06-08; HOD 06-78-06-07; HOD 06-77-18-30; HOD 06-77-17-27; Initial HOD 06-73-13-24] [Standard]

PREAMBLE

The Code of Ethics for the Physical Therapist (Code of Ethics) delineates the ethical obligations of all physical therapists as determined by the House of Delegates of the American Physical Therapy Association (APTA).

The purposes of this Code of Ethics are to:

1. Define the ethical principles that form the foundation of physical therapist practice in patient and client management, consultation, education, research, and administration.
2. Provide standards of behavior and performance that form the basis of professional accountability to the public.
3. Provide guidance for physical therapists facing ethical challenges, regardless of their professional roles and responsibilities.
4. Educate physical therapists, students, other health care professionals, regulators, and the public regarding the core values, ethical principles, and standards that guide the professional conduct of the physical therapist.
5. Establish the standards by which the American Physical Therapy Association can determine if a physical therapist has engaged in unethical conduct.

No code of ethics is exhaustive, nor can it address every situation. Physical therapists are encouraged to seek additional advice or consultation in instances where the guidance of the Code of Ethics may not be definitive. The APTA Guide for Professional Conduct and the APTA Core Values for the Physical Therapist and Physical Therapist Assistant provide additional guidance.

This Code of Ethics describes the desired behavior of physical therapists in their multiple roles (eg, management of patients and clients, consultation, education, research, and administration), addresses multiple aspects of ethical action (individual, organizational, and societal), and reflects the core values of the physical therapist (accountability, altruism, collaboration, compassion and caring, duty, excellence, integrity, and social responsibility). Throughout the document the primary core values that support specific principles are indicated in parentheses. Unless a specific role is indicated in the principle, the duties and obligations being delineated pertain to the five roles of the physical therapist. Fundamental to the Code of Ethics is the special obligation of physical therapists to empower, educate, and enable those with impairments, activity limitations, participation restrictions, and disabilities to facilitate greater independence, health, wellness, and enhanced quality of life.

PRINCIPLES

Principle #1: Physical therapists shall respect the inherent dignity and rights of all individuals.
(Core Values: Compassion and Caring, Integrity)

1A. Physical therapists shall act in a respectful manner toward each person regardless of age, gender, race, nationality, religion, ethnicity, social or economic status, sexual orientation, health condition, or disability.
1B. Physical therapists shall recognize their personal biases and shall not discriminate against others in physical therapist practice, consultation, education, research, and administration.

Principle #2: Physical therapists shall be trustworthy and compassionate in addressing the rights and needs of patients and clients.
(Core Values: Altruism, Collaboration, Compassion and Caring, Duty)

2A. Physical therapists shall adhere to the core values of the profession and shall act in the best interests of patients and clients over the interests of the physical therapist.
2B. Physical therapists shall provide physical therapist services with compassionate and caring behaviors that incorporate the individual and cultural differences of patients and clients.
2C. Physical therapists shall provide the information necessary to allow patients or their surrogates to make informed decisions about physical therapist care or participation in clinical research.
2D. Physical therapists shall collaborate with patients and clients to empower them in decisions about their health care.
2E. Physical therapists shall protect confidential patient and client information and may disclose confidential information to appropriate authorities only when allowed or as required by law.

Principle #3: Physical therapists shall be accountable for making sound professional judgments.
(Core Values: Collaboration, Duty, Excellence, Integrity)

3A. Physical therapists shall demonstrate independent and objective professional judgment in the patient's or client's best interest in all practice settings.

3B. Physical therapists shall demonstrate professional judgment informed by professional standards, evidence (including current literature and established best practice), practitioner experience, and patient and client values.

3C. Physical therapists shall make judgments within their scope of practice and level of expertise and shall communicate with, collaborate with, or refer to peers or other health care professionals when necessary.

3D. Physical therapists shall not engage in conflicts of interest that interfere with professional judgment.

3E. Physical therapists shall provide appropriate direction of and communication with physical therapistassistants and support personnel.

Principle #4: Physical therapists shall demonstrate integrity in their relationships with patients and clients, families, colleagues, students, research participants, other health care providers, employers, payers, and the public.
(Core Value: Integrity)

4A. Physical therapists shall provide truthful, accurate, and relevant information and shall not make misleading representations.

4B. Physical therapists shall not exploit persons over whom they have supervisory, evaluative or other authority (eg, patients/clients, students, supervisees, research participants, or employees).

4C. Physical therapists shall not engage in any sexual relationship with any of their patients and clients, supervisees, or students.

4D. Physical therapists shall not harass anyone verbally, physically, emotionally, or sexually.

4E. Physical therapists shall discourage misconduct by physical therapists, physical therapist assistants, and other health care professionals and, when appropriate, report illegal or unethical acts, including verbal, physical, emotional, or sexual harassment, to an appropriate authority with jurisdiction over the conduct.

4F. Physical therapists shall report suspected cases of abuse involving children or vulnerable adults to the appropriate authority, subject to law.

Principle #5: Physical therapists shall fulfill their legal and professional obligations.
(Core Values: Accountability, Duty, Social Responsibility)

5A. Physical therapists shall comply with applicable local, state, and federal laws and regulations.

5B. Physical therapists shall have primary responsibility for supervision of physical therapist assistants and support personnel.

5C. Physical therapists involved in research shall abide by accepted standards governing protection of research participants.

5D. Physical therapists shall encourage colleagues with physical, psychological, or substance-related impairments that may adversely impact their professional responsibilities to seek assistance or counsel.

5E. Physical therapists who have knowledge that a colleague is unable to perform their professional responsibilities with reasonable skill and safety shall report this information to the appropriate authority.

5F. Physical therapists shall provide notice and information about alternatives for obtaining care in the event the physical therapist terminates the provider relationship while the patient or client continues to need physical therapist services.

Principle #6: Physical therapists shall enhance their expertise through the lifelong acquisition and refinement of knowledge, skills, abilities, and professional behaviors.
(Core Value: Excellence)

6A. Physical therapists shall achieve and maintain professional competence.

6B. Physical therapists shall take responsibility for their professional development based on critical self-assessment and reflection on changes in physical therapist practice, education, health care delivery, and technology.

6C. Physical therapists shall evaluate the strength of evidence and applicability of content presented during professional development activities before integrating the content or techniques into practice.

6D. Physical therapists shall cultivate practice environments that support professional development, lifelong learning, and excellence.

Principle #7: Physical therapists shall promote organizational behaviors and business practices that benefit patients and clients and society.
(Core Values: Integrity, Accountability)

7A. Physical therapists shall promote practice environments that support autonomous and accountable professional judgments.

7B. Physical therapists shall seek remuneration as is deserved and reasonable for physical therapist services.

7C. Physical therapists shall not accept gifts or other considerations that influence or give an appearance of influencing their professional judgment.

7D. Physical therapists shall fully disclose any financial interest they have in products or services that they recommend to patients and clients.

7E. Physical therapists shall be aware of charges and shall ensure that documentation and coding for physical therapist services accurately reflect the nature and extent of the services provided.

7F. Physical therapists shall refrain from employment arrangements, or other arrangements, that prevent physical therapists from fulfilling professional obligations to patients and clients.

Principle #8: Physical therapists shall participate in efforts to meet the health needs of people locally, nationally, or globally.
(Core Value: Social Responsibility)

8A. Physical therapists shall provide pro bono physical therapist services or support organizations that meet the health needs of people who are economically disadvantaged, uninsured, and underinsured.

8B. Physical therapists shall advocate to reduce health disparities and health care inequities, improve access to health care services, and address the health, wellness, and preventive health care needs of people.

8C. Physical therapists shall be responsible stewards of health care resources and shall avoid overutilization or under-utilization of physical therapist services.

8D. Physical therapists shall educate members of the public about the benefits of physical therapy and the unique role of the physical therapist.

Explanation of Reference Numbers:

HOD P00-00-00-00 stands for House of Delegates/month/year/page/vote in the House of Delegates minutes; the "P" indicates that it is a position (see below). For example, HOD P06-17-05-04 means that this position can be found in the June 2017 House of Delegates minutes on Page 5 and that it was Vote 4.

P: Position | S: Standard | G: Guideline | Y: Policy | R: Procedure
Last Updated: 8/12/2020
Contact: nationalgovernance@apta.org

Standards of Ethical Conduct for the Physical Therapist Assistant

HOD S06-20-31-26 [Amended HOD S06-19-47-68; HOD S06-09-20-18; HOD S06-00-13-24; HOD 06-91-06-07; Initial HOD 06-82-04-08] [Standard]

PREAMBLE

The Standards of Ethical Conduct for the Physical Therapist Assistant (Standards of Ethical Conduct) delineate the ethical obligations of all physical therapist assistants as determined by the House of Delegates of the American Physical Therapy Association (APTA). The Standards of Ethical Conduct provide a foundation for conduct to which all physical therapist assistants shall adhere. Physical therapist assistants are guided by a set of core values (accountability, altruism, collaboration, compassion and caring, duty, excellence, integrity, and social responsibility). Throughout the document the primary core values that support specific principles are indicated in parentheses. Fundamental to the Standards of Ethical Conduct is the special obligation of physical therapist assistants to enable patients and clients to achieve greater independence, health and wellness, and enhanced quality of life.

No document that delineates ethical standards can address every situation. Physical therapist assistants are encouraged to seek additional advice or consultation in instances where the guidance of the Standards of Ethical Conduct may not be definitive. The APTA Guide for Conduct of the Physical Therapist Assistant and the APTA Core Values for the Physical Therapist and Physical Therapist Assistant provide additional guidance.

Standards

Standard #1: Physical therapist assistants shall respect the inherent dignity, and rights, of all individuals.
(Core Values: Compassion and Caring, Integrity)

1A. Physical therapist assistants shall act in a respectful manner toward each person regardless of age, gender, race, nationality, religion, ethnicity, social or economic status, sexual orientation, health condition, or disability.

1B. Physical therapist assistants shall recognize their personal biases and shall not discriminate against others in the provision of physical therapist services.

Standard #2: Physical therapist assistants shall be trustworthy and compassionate in addressing the rights and needs of patients and clients.
(Core Values: Altruism, Collaboration, Compassion and Caring, Duty)

2A. Physical therapist assistants shall act in the best interests of patients and clients over the interests of the physical therapist assistant.

2B. Physical therapist assistants shall provide physical therapist interventions with compassionate and caring behaviors that incorporate the individual and cultural differences of patients and clients.

2C. Physical therapist assistants shall provide patients and clients with information regarding the interventions they provide.

2D. Physical therapist assistants shall protect confidential patient and client information and, in collaboration with the physical therapist, may disclose confidential information to appropriate authorities only when allowed or as required by law.

Standard #3: Physical therapist assistants shall make sound decisions in collaboration with the physical therapist and within the boundaries established by laws and regulations.
(Core Values: Collaboration, Duty, Excellence, Integrity)

3A. Physical therapist assistants shall make objective decisions in the patient's or client's best interest in all practice settings.

3B. Physical therapist assistants shall be guided by information about best practice regarding physical therapist interventions.

3C. Physical therapist assistants shall make decisions based upon their level of competence and consistent with patient and client values.

3D. Physical therapist assistants shall not engage in conflicts of interest that interfere with making sound decisions.

3E. Physical therapist assistants shall provide physical therapist services under the direction and supervision of a physical therapist and shall communicate with the physical therapist when patient or client status requires modifications to the established plan of care.

Standard #4: Physical therapist assistants shall demonstrate integrity in their relationships with patients and clients, families, colleagues, students, research participants other health care providers, employers, payers, and the public.
(Core Value: Integrity)

4A. Physical therapist assistants shall provide truthful, accurate, and relevant information and shall not make misleading representations.

4B. Physical therapist assistants shall not exploit persons over whom they have supervisory, evaluative or other authority (eg, patients and clients, students, supervisees, research participants, or employees).

4C. Physical therapist assistants shall not engage in any sexual relationship with any of their patients and clients, supervisees, or students.

4D. Physical therapist assistants shall not harass anyone verbally, physically, emotionally, or sexually.

4E. Physical therapist assistants shall discourage misconduct by physical therapists, physical therapist assistants, and other health care professionals and, when appropriate, report illegal or unethical acts, including verbal, physical, emotional, or sexual harassment, to an appropriate authority with jurisdiction over the conduct.

4F. Physical therapist assistants shall report suspected cases of abuse involving children or vulnerable adults to the appropriate authority, subject to law.

Standard #5: Physical therapist assistants shall fulfill their legal and ethical obligations.
(Core Values: Accountability, Duty, Social Responsibility)

5A. Physical therapist assistants shall comply with applicable local, state, and federal laws and regulations.

5B. Physical therapist assistants shall support the supervisory role of the physical therapist to ensure quality care and promote patient and client safety.

5C. Physical therapist assistants involved in research shall abide by accepted standards governing protection of research participants.

5D. Physical therapist assistants shall encourage colleagues with physical, psychological, or substance- related impairments that may adversely impact their professional responsibilities to seek assistance or counsel.

5E. Physical therapist assistants who have knowledge that a colleague is unable to perform their professional responsibilities with reasonable skill and safety shall report this information to the appropriate authority.

Standard #6: Physical therapist assistants shall enhance their competence through the lifelong acquisition and refinement of knowledge, skills, and abilities.
(Core Value: Excellence)

6A. Physical therapist assistants shall achieve and maintain clinical competence.

6B. Physical therapist assistants shall engage in lifelong learning consistent with changes in their roles and responsibilities and advances in the practice of physical therapy.

6C. Physical therapist assistants shall support practice environments that support career development and lifelong learning.

Standard #7: Physical therapist assistants shall support organizational behaviors and business practices that benefit patients and clients and society.
(Core Values: Integrity, Accountability)

7A. Physical therapist assistants shall promote work environments that support ethical and accountable decision-making.

7B. Physical therapist assistants shall not accept gifts or other considerations that influence or give an appearance of influencing their decisions.

7C. Physical therapist assistants shall fully disclose any financial interest they have in products or services that they recommend to patients and clients.

7D. Physical therapist assistants shall ensure that documentation for their interventions accurately reflects the nature and extent of the services provided.

7E. Physical therapist assistants shall refrain from employment arrangements, or other arrangements, that prevent physical therapist assistants from fulfilling ethical obligations to patients and clients.

Standard #8: Physical therapist assistants shall participate in efforts to meet the health needs of people locally, nationally, or globally.
(Core Value: Social Responsibility)

8A. Physical therapist assistants shall support organizations that meet the health needs of people who are economically disadvantaged, uninsured, and underinsured.

8B. Physical therapist assistants shall advocate for people with impairments, activity limitations, participation restrictions, and disabilities in order to promote their participation in community and society.

8C. Physical therapist assistants shall be responsible stewards of health care resources by collaborating with physical therapists in order to avoid overutilization or underutilization of physical therapist services.

8D. Physical therapist assistants shall educate members of the public about the benefits of physical therapy.

Explanation of Reference Numbers:

HOD P00-00-00-00 stands for House of Delegates/month/year/page/vote in the House of Delegates minutes; the "P" indicates that it is a position (see below). For example, HOD P06-17-05-04 means that this position can be found in the June 2017 House of Delegates minutes on Page 5 and that it was Vote 4.

P: Position | S: Standard | G: Guideline | Y: Policy | R: Procedure
Last Updated: 8/12/2020
Contact: nationalgovernance@apta.org

Answers to Ideas to Consider

CHAPTER 1

1. c. Organizational priorities and financial pressures affect everyday decisions.
2. d. Trust.
3. a. Patients are vulnerable.
4. b. A willingness to partner responsibly with their provider.
5. a. Being kind.
6. c. Doing no harm.
7. a. Fairness.
8. d. Truthfulness founded on a respect for persons.
9. a. Compromise your integrity.
10. b. The capacity to take moral action responsibly in the face of adversity.
11. d. Ethically but illegally.

CHAPTER 2

1. b. Dynamic.
2. a. All have a guidance document like a Code of Ethics.
3. e. All of the above are true.

CHAPTER 3

1. f. All of the above.
2. b. Competence.
3. b. Survival skills.

CHAPTER 4

1. b. PTs are facing more ethical situations.
2. c. Guidance for the physical therapist assistant.
3. a. All physical therapists.
4. d. Every PT must take responsibility for all aspects of their practice.

CHAPTER 5

1. b. All therapists in all settings.
2. a. Critical self-reflection.
3. c. System failures.

CHAPTER 6

1. b. An ethical dilemma.
2. d. Moral courage.
3. b. Moral judgment.
4. d. An ethical silence.
5. b. Rule based.
6. c. Ends based.
7. a. Implement, evaluate, and reassess.

CHAPTER 7

1. b. Telecommunication.
2. c. A location for treatment.
3. c. A and B.

References

Aicardi C, DelSalvio L, Dove E, et al. Emerging ethical issues regarding digital health data. On the world medical association draft declaration of ethical considerations regarding health databases and biobanks. *Croat Med J*. 2016;57(2):207-213.

Airth-Kindree NM, Kirkhorn LE. Ethical grand rounds: teaching ethics at the point of care. *Nurs Educ Perspect*. 2016;37(1):48-50.

American Physical Therapy Association (APTA). Core Documents: Code of Ethics. 2017a. Available at APTA.org. Accessed December 1, 2022.

American Physical Therapy Association (APTA). Core Documents: Standards of Ethical Conduct. 2017b. Available at APTA.org. Accessed December 1, 2022.

American Physical Therapy Association (APTA). DPT degree PT in Motion News: July 10, 2014. Available at APTA.org. Accessed December 1, 2022.

American Telehealth Association 2023. Available at https://www.americantelemed.org. Accessed September 15, 2023.

Australian Council of Professions. Available at https://www.professions.org.au.

Avey JB, Avolino BJ, Crossley CD, et al. Psychological ownership, theoretical extensions, measurement, and relation to work outcomes. *J Organ Behav*. 2009;30:173-181.

Avolio BJ, Reichard RJ, Hannah ST, et al. 100 years of leadership intervention studies: a meta-analysis. *Leadersh Q*. 2009;20:764-784.

Badawi A. Boundaries in therapeutic practice. *J Aust Trad Med Soc*. 2016;22(21):90-93.

Balak N, Broekman M, Mathiesen T. Ethics in contemporary health care management and medical education. *J Eval Clin Pract*. 2020;26:699-706.

Barnett J, Behnke S, Rosenthal S, et al. In case of ethical dilemma, break glass: Commentary on ethical decision making in practice. *Prof Psychol Res Pr*. 2005;38(1):7-12.

Baum N. Balancing your personal and professional lives. *Ochsner J*. 2008;8(4):160-162.

Beauchamp TL, Childress JF. *Principles of Biomedical Ethics*. 5th ed. New York, NY: Oxford University Press; 2001:228.

Bernard D. Vulnerability and trustworthiness. *Camb Q Healthc Ethics*. 2016;25(2):288-300.

Bismark MM, Studdert DM, Morton K, Paterson R, Spittal MJ, Taouk Y. Sexual misconduct by health professionals in Australia 2011-2016: a retrospective analysis of notifications to health regulators. *Med J Aust*. 2020;213(5):218-224.

Borges LM, Barnes SM, Farnsworth JK, Bahraini NH, Brenner LA. A commentary on moral injury among health care providers during the COVID-19 pandemic. *Psychol Trauma*. 2020;12(S1):S138-S140.

Brecke F, Garcia S. *Training Methodology for Logistic Decision-Making* (No. AI/HR-TP-1995-0098). Brooks AFB, TX: United States Air Force; 1995.

Brody H, Doukas D. Professionalism: A framework to guide medical education. *Med Educ*. 2014;48(10):980-987.

Caldicott C, D'Oronzio J. Ethics remediation, rehabilitation and recommitment to medical professionalism: A programmatic approach. *Ethics Behav.* 2014;25(4):279-296.

Commission Accreditation of Physical Therapy Education (CAPTE) Programs 2016. Available at https://www.capteonline.org. Accessed December 1, 2022.

Cheshire WP. Telemedicine and the ethics of medical care at a distance. *Ethics and Medicine.* 2017;33:2.

CNA-HPSO. Physical therapy professional liability exposures: 2020 claim report. Available at https://www.hpso.com/getmedia/843bca04-caa8-47aa-be5d-52d307495944/physical-therapy-claim-report-fourth-edition.pdf- claim-report-. Accessed December 11, 2022.

Creuss SR, Johnston S, Creuss R. "Profession" a working definition for medical educators. *Teach Learn Med.* 2004;16(1).

Cruess SR. Professionalism and medicine's social contract with society. *Clin Orthop Relat Res.* 2006;449:170-176.

Dale S. How do you make ethical decisions. *Ther Today.* 2016;27(6):36-39.

Dar U, Kahn Y. Self reported academic misconduct among medical students: perception and prevalence. *ScientificWorldJournal.* 2021:1-8.

Dean W, Talbot S, Dean A. Reframing clinician Distress: moral injury not burnout. *Fed Pract.* 2019;36(9):400-402.

deOliveira V, Santos M, Jacinto A, et al. Why medical schools are tolerant of unethical behavior. *Ann Fam Med.* 2015;13(2):176-180.

Dove L. Ethics training for the alcohol, drug abuse professional. *Alcohol Treat Q.* 1995;12(4):19-38.

Drumwright M. Behavioral ethics and teaching ethical decision making. *DSJIE.* 2015;13(3):431-458.

Dubois JM, Anderson EE, Chibnall JT, et al. Preventing egregious ethical violations in medical practice, evidence-informed recommendations from a multidisciplinary working group. *J Med Reg.* 2018;104(4):23-31.

Dubois JM, Walsh HA, Chibnall JT, et al. Sexual violation of patients by physicians: a mixed-methods, exploratory analysis of 101 cases. *Sexual Abuse.* 2019;31(5) 503-523.

Edelstein L. The Hippocratic oath: text, translation and interpretation. In: Temkin O, Temkin CL, eds. *Ancient Medicine: Selected Papers of Ludwig Edelstein.* Baltimore, MD: Johns Hopkins Press; 1967:3-64.

Elger B, Harding T. Terminally ill patients and Jehovah's witnesses teaching acceptance of patients' refusals of vital treatments. *Med Educ.* 2002;36(5):479-488.

Evetts J. Sociological analysis of professionalism: past, present and future. *Comp Sociol.* 2011;10:1-37.

Ford A. Accountability for reasonableness: the relevance, or not of exceptionality in resource allocation. *Health Care Philos.* 2015;18(2):217-227.

FSBPT. *Model Practice Act.* 6th ed.

FSMB. *Physician Sexual Misconduct: Report and Recommendations of the FSMB Workgroup on Physician Sexual Misconduct.* May 2020.

Gabard DL, Martin MW. *Physical Therapy Ethics.* Philadelphia, PA: Davis; 2003.

Gallagher CT, Thaci J, Saadalla G, et al. Disciplinary action against UK health professionals for sexual misconduct: a matter of reputational damage or public safety? *J Med Regul.* 2021;107(4):7-16.

Goud NH. Courage: its nature and development. *J Humanist Couns Educ Dev.* 2005; 44:102-116.

Guccione A. Ethical issues in physical therapy practice: a survey of physical therapists in New England. *Phys Ther.* 1980;60(10):1264.

Hagan JB. Stem cells: New frontiers in science and ethics. *Curr Rev Acad Libr.* 2013; 50(5):900-902.

Handelsman M. Problems with ethics training by osmosis. *Prof Psychol Res Pr.* 1986; 17:371-372.

Hannah ST, Avolio BJ, Luthans F, et al. Leadership efficacy: Review and future directions. *Leadership Q.* 2008;19:669-692.

Hannah ST, Avolio BJ, May DR. Moral maturation and moral conation: A capacity approach to explaining moral thought and action. *Acad Manag Rev.* 2011a. Available at http://www.ioatwork.com/the-makings-of-morality-the-factors-behind-ethical-behavior/. Accessed September 18, 2012.

Hannah ST, Avolio BJ, Walumbwa FO. Relationships between authentic leadership, moral courage, and ethical and pro-social behaviors. *Bus Ethics Q.* 2011b;226-240.

Hannah ST, Avolio BJ. Moral potency: building the capacity for character-based leadership. *Consulting Psychol J.* 2010;62:291-310.

Hannah ST, Woolfolk L, Lord RG. Leader self-structure: a framework for positive leadership. *J Organ Behav.* 2009;30:269-290.

Hartman M, Catlin A, Lasserman D, et al. U.S. health spending by age, selected years through 2004. *Health Aff.* 2008;27:1-12.

Harvard Law Review. The Hart Fuller Debate. 1958.

Hightower BB, Klinker JF. When ethics and policy collide. *J Cases Educ Leadersh.* 2012; 15(2):103-111.

Hren D, Marusic M, Marusic A. Regression of moral reasoning during medical education: Combined design study to evaluate the effect of clinical study years. *PLoS One.* 2011;6(3).

Hudon A, Drolet MJ, Williams-Jones B. Ethical issues raised by private practice physiotherapy are more diverse than first meets the eye: recommendations from a literature review. *Physiother Can.* 2015;67(2):124-132

Janoff-Bulman R, Sheikh S, Hepp S. Proscriptive versus prescriptive morality: Two faces of moral regulation. *J Pers Soc Psychol.* 2009;96:521-537.

Juengst E, McGowan M, Fishman J, et al. From personalized to precision medicine: The ethical and social implications of rhetorical reform in genomic medicine. *Hastings Cent Rep.* 2016;46(5):21-33.

Kaiser Foundation Fact Sheet: Medicare Beneficiaries. 2020.

Kaldjian L, Rosenbaum M, Shinkunas L, et al. Through students' eyes: Ethical and professional issues identified by third-year medical students during clerkships. *J Med Issues.* 2013;38:130-132.

Kearney G, Penque S. Ethics of everyday decision making. *Nurs Manag.* 2012;19(1) 32-36.

Keehan S, Sisko A, Truffer C, et al. Health spending projections through 2017: The baby-boom generation is coming to Medicare. *Health Aff.* 2008;27(2):145-155.

Kidder RM. *How Good People Make Tough Choices: Resolving the Dilemmas of Ethical Living.* New York, NY: Morrow; 1996.

Kilic Y, Chauhan D, Avery P, et al. The public's attitude towards doctors' use of Twitter and perceived professionalism: an exploratory study. *Clin Med.* 2021;21(5):e475-e479.

King PA, Chaudhry H, Staz M. State medical board recommendations for stronger approaches to sexual misconduct by physicians. *JAMA*. 2021;325(16):1609-1610.

Kirsch N. Ethical decision making: terminology and context. *PT Magaz Phys Ther*. 2006;14(2):38-40.

Kirsch N. Ethics in practice. *PT Magaz Phys Ther*. Ahead of print. February 2017.

Kirsch N. *The Level at Which Practicing Physical Therapists Make Ethical Decisions*. Ann Arbor, MI: UMI Dissertation Services; 2003:100.

Knapp S, Handelsman M, Gottlieb M, et al. The dark side of professional ethics. *Prof Psychol Res Pr*. 2013a;44(6):371-377.

Knapp S, Vandecreek L, Handelsman M, et al. Professional decisions and behaviors on the ethical rim. *Prof Psychol Res Pr*. 2013b;44(6) 378-383.

Kornblau BL, Starling SP. *Ethics in Rehabilitation: A Clinical Perspective*. Thorofare, NJ: Slack; 2000.

Lanier J, W, Hasseman C, Revised by Dzubak J. Basics of professional boundaries and sexual misconduct for nurses. *Ohio Nurs Rev*. 2018;93(4):14-18.

Leeuwenburgh-Pronk W, Miller-Smith L, Forman V, et al. Are we allowed to discontinue medical treatment in this child. *Pediatrics*. 2015;135(3):545-549.

Mansbach A, Melzer I, Bachner YG. Blowing the whistle to protect a patient: A comparison between physiotherapy students and physiotherapists. *Physiotherapy*. 2012;98(4): 307-312.

Marques J. Ethics: walking the talk. *JQP*. 2012;34(6):4-7.

Maslach C, Jackson S, Leitner M. *Maslach Burnout Inventory Manual*. 3rd ed. Palo Alto, CA: Consulting Psychologists Press; 1996.

McCarthy J, Gastmans C. Moral distress: a review of the argument based nursing ethics literature. *Nurs Ethics*. 2015;22(1):131-152.

McWilliams M, Meara E, Zaslavsky A, et al. Use of health services by previously uninsured medicare beneficiaries. *N Engl J Med*. 2007;357(2):143-153.

Means J, Kodner I, Brown D, et al. Sharing clinical photographs: patient rights, professional ethics, and institutional responsibilities. *Bull Am Coll Surg*. 2015;100(10):17-22.

Medpac: Report to the Congress: Medicare and the Health Care Delivery System. June, 2015. Available at https://www.medpac.gov/wp-content/uploads/import_data/scrape_files/docs/default-source/reports/chapter-2-the-next-generation-of-medicare-beneficiaries-june-2015-report-.pdf. Accessed December 22, 2022.

Miles S, Prasad S. Medical ethics in school football. *Am J Bioeth*. 2016;16(1):6-10.

Morley G, Grady C, McCarthy J, Ulrich C. Covid-19: Ethical challenges for nurses. *Hastings Cent Rep*. 2020;50(3):35-39.

Morris K, Simpkins W, Hasseman C. Basics of professional boundaries and sexual misconduct for nurses. *Ohio Nurs Rev*. 2018;93(4):14-18.

Mourad F, Patuzzo A, Tenci A, et al. Giuseppe, Management of whiplash-associated disorder in the Italian emergency department: the feasibility of an evidence-based continuous professional development course provided by physiotherapists. *Disabil Rehabil*. 2022;44(10):2123-2130.

Murrell C. The failure of medical education to develop moral reasoning in medical students. *Int J Med Educ*. 2014;5:219-225.

Naamanka K, Suhonen R, Puukka P, Tolvanen A, Leino-Kilpi H. Self evaluated ethical competence of a practicing physiotherapist: a national study in Finland. *BMC Med Ethics*. 2020;21(1):43.

Nebeker C, Bartlett Ellis R, Torous J. CORE tools. Digital health decision making framework and checklist designed for researchers. 2018. Available at https://recode.health/dmcheck-list. Accessed August 5, 2022.

Nebeker C, Bartlett Ellis RJ, Torous J. Development of a decision-making checklist tool to support technology selection in digital health research. *Transl Behav Med.* 2020;10(4):1004-1015.

Nebeker C, Torous J, Bartlett Ellis RJ. Building the case for actionable ethics in digital health research supported by artificial intelligence. *BMC Med.* 2019;17(1):1-7.

Newkrug E, Lovell C, Parker RJ. Employing ethical codes and decision-making models: A developmental process. *Couns Values.* 1996;40(2):98-106.

Nijhof A, Wilderom C, Oost M. Professional and institutional morality: Building ethics programmes on the dual loyalty of academic professionals. *Ethics and Education.* 2012;7(1):91-109.

O'Fallon MJ, Butterfield KD. A review of the empirical ethical decision-making literature: 1996–2003. *J Bus Ethics.* 2005;59:375-413.

Oeffner J. From the playground to the workplace, managing bullying in health care. APTA Combined Sections meeting. 2014.

Osswald S, Greitemeyer T, Fischer P, et al. What is moral courage? Definition, explication and classification of a complex construct. In: Pury C, Lopez S, eds. *The Psychology of Courage: Modern Research on an Ancient Virtue.* American Psychological Association; 2009:94-120.

Pagoto S, Nebeker C. How scientists can take the lead in establishing ethical practices for social media research. *J Am Med Infor Assoc.* 2019;26(4):311-313.

Pantic N, Wubbels T. Teachers' moral values and their interpersonal relationships with students and cultural competence. *Teach Teach Educ.* 2012;28:451-460.

Pasztor J. What is ethics anyway? *JFSP.* 2015;69(6):30-32.

Pellegrino E. The metamorphosis of medical ethics: A 30-year retrospective. *JAMA.* 1993;269(9):1158-1162.

Pellegrino E. The origins and evolution of bioethics: Some personal reflections. *Kennedy Inst Ethics J.* 1999;9(1):73-88.

Phipps E, True G, Harris D, et al. Approaching the end of life: Attitudes, preferences, and behaviors of African-American and white patients and their family caregivers. *J Clin Oncol.* 2003;21(3):549-554.

Price D. Social Contract Table Update: Creuss and Creuss. 2015.

Professional Standards Councils: Definition from Professions Australia website https://www.professions.org.au/what-is-a-professional/. Accessed December 2022.

Pruthi R. Moral Injury and how it applies to physicians. *Urology Times.* May 2019.

Queensland Nurse. Mandatory reporting your obligations. *Queensland Nurse.* 2011;(5):34-35.

Quigley M. Evidence and ethics: one more into the fray. *J Med Ethics.* 2015;41(10):793-794.

Rate CR, Clarke JA, Lindsay DR, et al. Implicit theories of courage. *J Posit Psychol.* 2007;2:80-98.

Rawson J, Thompson N, Sostre G, et al. The cost of disruptive and unprofessional behaviors in health care. *Acad Radiol.* 2013;20(9):1074-1076.

Reuben D, Levy-Storms L, Yee M. Disciplinary split: a threat to geriatrics interdisciplinary team training. *J Am Geriatr Soc.* 2004;52:10.

Rosenthal SA, Pittinsky TL, Purvin DM, et al. National Leadership Index 2007: a national study of confidence in leadership. In: John F, ed. *Center for Public Leadership*. Cambridge, MA: Kennedy School of Government, Harvard University; 2007.

Schaubroeck J, Hannah ST, Avolio BJ, et al. Excellence in Character and Ethical Leadership (EXCEL) study. Center for the army profession and ethics technical report 2010-01. West Point, NY: U.S. Army; 2010.

Scott R. *Professional Ethics: A Guide for Rehabilitation Professionals*. New York, NY: Mosby; 1998.

Shay J. Moral injury. *Psychoanal Psychol*. 2014;31(2):182-191. https://doi.org/10.1037/a0036090.

Shih S, Gerrard P, Goldstein R, et al. Functional status outperforms comorbidities in predicting acute care readmissions in medically complex patients. *J Gen Med*. 2015;30(11):1688-1695.

Sisola S. Patient vulnerability: ethical considerations for physical therapists. *PT Magazine*. 2003;11(7):46-50.

Smith T, McGuire J, Abbott D, et al. Clinical ethical decision making: an investigation of the rationales used to justify doing less than one believes one should. *Prof Psychol*. 1991;22(3):235-239.

Sokol D. Once a month, or the secret to raising the status of medical ethics. *BMJ*. 2015; 41(10):854-858.

Stahl B, Coeckelbergh M. Ethics of healthcare robotics: towards responsible research and innovation. *Rob Auton Syst*. 2016;86:152-161.

Starr KT. Reporting a physician colleague for unsafe practice: what's the law? *Nursing*. 2019;46(2):14.

Starr L. A 10 year ban for breaching professional boundaries: crossing professional boundaries is a breach of trust-particularly when this involves sexual misconduct. *Aust Nurs Midwifery J*. 2020;27(1):21.

Strudwick K, Martin R, Coombes F, Bell A, Martin-Khan M, Russell T. Trevor Higher quality of care in emergency departments with physiotherapy service models. *Emerg Med Australas*. 2022;34(2):209-222.

Strum A, Edwards I, Fryer CE, Roth R. (Almost) 50 shades of an ethical situation-international physiotherapists' experiences of everyday ethics: A qualitative analysis. *Physiother Theory Pract*. 2023;39(2):351-368. doi:10.1080/09593985.2021.2015812. Epub 2022 Jan 4.

Sugarman J. *Twenty Common Problems: Ethics in Primary Care*. New York, NY: McGraw-Hill; 2000.

Sujdak M, Birgitta N. Good ethics begin with good facts. *Am J Bioeth*. 2016;16(7):66-68.

SullivanLuallin Group. C.L.E.A.R. protocol for patient satisfaction. Available at http://www.sullivanluallingroup.com/patient-experience-consulting/five-star-service-is-clear-dvd/. Accessed June 4, 2017.

Sutherland-Smith W, Saltmarsh S. In search of an ethical university. *Ethics and Education*. 2011;6(3):213-215.

Swisher L, Arslanian L, Davis C. The realm-individual process-situation (RIPS) model of ethical decision making. *HPA Resource*. 2005;5(3):1, 3-8.

Taylor N. Nonsurgical management of osteoarthritis knee pain in the older adult. *Clin Geriatr Med*. 2017;33(1):41-51.

Tenbrunsel AE, Messick DM. Ethical fading: The role of self-deception in unethical behavior. *Soc Justice Res.* 2008;17:223-236.

Tenbrunsel AE, Smith-Crowe K. Ethical decision-making: where we've been and where we're going. *Acad Manag Annals.* 2008;2:545-607.

Tenery RM. Medical ethics: medical etiquette. *JAMA.* 2016; 315(12):1291.

Thorpe K, Howard D. The rise in spending among medicare beneficiaries: the role of chronic disease prevalence and changes in treatment intensity. *Health Aff.* 2006;25(5):378-388.

Tymchuk A, Drapkin R, Major-Kingsley S, et al. Ethical decision-making and psychologists' attitudes toward training in ethics. *Prof Psychol Res Pr.* 1982;13(3):412-421.

Valente SM, Saunders JM. Oncology nurses' difficulties with suicide. *Med Law.* 2000;19(4):793-814.

Veatch RM. *The Basics of Bioethics.* 4th ed. Routledge Press; 2016.

Wells DM, Lehavot K, Isaac ML. Sounding off on social media: the ethics of patient storytelling in the modern era. *Acad Med.* 2015;90(8):1015-1019.

Welsh D, Ordonez L. Conscience without cognition: the effects of subconscious priming on ethical behavior. *Acad Manag J.* 2014;57(3):723-742.

Wojcicki P, Drozdowski P. In utero surgery—Current state of the art: Part 1. *Med Sci Monit.* 2010;16(11):237-244.

Xu Z, Ma H. How can a deontological decision lead to moral behavior? The moderating role of moral identity. *J Bus Ethics.* 2016;37(3) 537-549.

Zviliac JE, Toriscelli TA, Merrick WS, et al. Isokinetic concentric quadriceps and hamstring normative data for elite collegiate American football players participating in the NFL scouting combine. *J Strength Cond Res.* 2014;28:875.

Index

Index